Pilates Evolution
The 21st Century

by Joseph H. Pilates
and
Judd Robbins and Lin Van Heuit-Robbins

Pilates Evolution
The 21st Century

by Joseph H. Pilates
and
Judd Robbins and Lin Van Heuit-Robbins

Published by Presentation Dynamics
949-666-5030
http://www.JosephPilates.org
ISBN 13: 978-1-928564-91-1
Library of Congress Control Number: 2012935680

Photographs of:
Joseph H. Pilates at sixty
Judd Robbins at sixty-six
Lin Van Heuit-Robbins at fifty-nine

Dedications

Judd Robbins: To my mother, Betty Robbins, for a lifetime of unlimited encouragement and support.

Lin Van Heuit-Robbins: To my favorite daughter Alix, my favorite son Greg, my favorite younger stepson Eli, my favorite older stepson Josh, and the chickens.

Photographer: Jo Ann Weisel

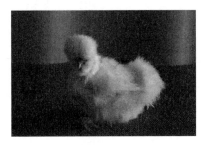

Chicken: Barbie

INTRODUCTION to Pilates Evolution

by Judd Robbins and Lin Van Heuit-Robbins

Joseph Pilates preached the benefits of a perfect balance of body and mind. He also followed his own teachings. He coupled his background in gymnastics and martial arts with a keen analytical approach to body mechanics, posture, and correct breathing. All of these fundamentals appealed to us intellectually. Once we experienced his recommendations for exercises, postural modifications and breathing mechanisms, we truly began to feel like converts.

Our own background in fitness and athletics began years ago with competitive high school and college athletics. Lin was a gymnast and Judd was a tennis and squash player. After college, Lin went on to design and teach a variety of programs in aerobics, stretching and flexibility, and weight training. She studied advanced methodologies in exercise physiology while obtaining a Masters Degree at the University of California at Berkeley. She also holds certifications in group fitness training and personal training from the American Council on Exercise (ACE). Beyond those credentials, she has been a reviewer for the ACE correspondence accreditation committee.

Judd combines a degree in physics with advanced degrees from the University of Michigan and the University of California at Berkeley, and has developed his own analytical and experiential approach to exercise. He was a racquetball pro in the late '70s, has earned a 3rd degree black belt in jujitsu plus a group fitness certification from the American Council on Exercise. He has been developing and teaching Pilates, yoga, and various exercise classes for many years. Both Lin and Judd are certified by the PhysicalMind Institute in New York City in the matwork originally developed by Joseph and Clara Pilates.

There are many excellent books in the field of health, exercise, and fitness. We've studied and use the principles offered in many of them, from yoga to stretching to strength training. In our current classes, we have incorporated the latest innovations in Pilates training, both with and without props, in standing, sitting, and lying down positions. We strongly believe that Joseph Pilates created a truly effective combination of strengthening and stretching that can work well for virtually everybody. With the right instruction and guidance, some or all of Pilates' recommendations can demonstrably improve anybody's health and fitness levels.

This new book includes Joseph Pilates' original 1936 book of fitness principles entitled *Your Health*, as well as his 1945 work entitled *Return to Life through Contrology*. We own and authorize translations and reprints of his original writings, as well as this new combination book, in foreign languages around the world. This book, as well as his original works which we publish, retain the original photographs and step-by-step poses and accompanying instructions. While some of the latest research in the fitness world might suggest caution when performing some of these poses and exercises, the overall program of exercises developed at the turn of the 20th Century remains astoundingly effective and beneficial for fitness enthusiasts in the 21st Century.

As with all exercise programs, you should consult your doctor before following any or all of the exercises and poses presented in this book. The overall impact of Joseph Pilates' exercises can be extraordinarily beneficial to anyone suffering from a variety of physical weaknesses. However, the exercises are most effective when presented to beginners by a trainer who has studied Pilates' original matwork instructions as well as the fundamental physiological and biomechanical aspects of the body that are so analytically coordinated into the exercises by Joseph Pilates. In particular, the latest evolutionary training techniques presented in this new work, *Pilates Evolution*, require instructors who are knowledgeable in the application of Pilates' principles to recent developments in fitness.

TABLE of CONTENTS
for
Pilates Evolution - The 21st Century

Part I – Your Health (Original Edition).................9

Introducing Part I and Pilates' View of Your Health 10

Chapter 1: A Grave Situation...21

Chapter 2: Health — A Normal-Natural Condition....................................27

Chapter 3: Dreadful Conditions 33

Chapter 4: Heading Downward 38

Chapter 5: Common Sense Remedies for Common Human Ills! 44

Chapter 6: "Contrology" 52

Chapter 7: "Balance of Body and Mind"..56

Chapter 8: First Educate the Child! 57

Chapter 9: Proved Facts! 64

Chapter 10: New Style Beds and Chairs...71

Part II – Contrology (Original Edition)..................81

Introducing Part II and Fitness Principles Evolved from Contrology 82
Return to Life through Contrology – Original Edition 85
Basic Fundamentals of a Natural Physical Education............................95
   Civilization Impairs Physical Fitness 95
   Contrology Restores Physical Fitness 98
   Guiding Principles of Contrology... 100
   Bodily House-cleaning with Blood Circulation................................. 101
   Results of Contrology 110
The Original Exercises...**113**
   1. The Hundred... 114
   2. The Roll Up 116
   3. The Roll-Over With Legs Spread (Both Ways).................. 118
   4. The One Leg Circle (Both Ways)..................................... 120
   5. Rolling Back 122
   6. The One Leg Stretch 124
   7. The Double Leg Stretch.. 126
   8. The Spine Stretch 128
   9. Rocker With Open Legs 130
   10. The Cork-Screw 132
   11. The Saw 134
   12. The Swan-Dive 136
   13. The One Leg Kick... 138
   14. The Double Kick... 140
   15. The Neck Pull 142
   16. The Scissors... 144
   17. The Bicycle 146
   18. The Shoulder Bridge 148
   19. The Spine Twist 150
   20. The Jack Knife 152
   21. The Side Kick 154
   22. The Teaser 156
   23. The Hip Twist With Stretched Arms............................... 158
   24. Swimming.. 160
   25. The Leg-Pull — Front.. 162
   26. The Leg-Pull 164
   27. The Side Kick Kneeling 166
   28. The Side Bend.. 168
   29. The Boomerang.. 170
   30. The Seal... 172
   31. The Crab 174
   32. The Rocking 176
   33. The Control Balance 178
   34. The Push Up 180

Part III – 21st Century Pilates Evolution 183

Introduction to Evolutionary Developments 187

Chapter 1: Pilates Magic Circle 191

Chapter 2: Weights..197

Chapter 3: Seated Pilates 203

Chapter 4: Mini Stability Ball..209

Chapter 5: Elastic Resistance 215

Chapter 6: Standing Work 221

Chapter 7: Circular Work 227

Chapter 8: 'Unstable' Surfaces' 233

Chapter 9: Fusion Classes 239

Chapter 10: Sports Specific Pilates 245

Appendix A: Glossary of Pilates' terms...................................251

Appendix B: Index 255

Part I

1934 Edition of

Joseph Pilates'
Your Health

Introducing Part I and Pilates' View of Your Health

Joseph Pilates was a man with very strong opinions. In 1934, he published his first book, *Your Health*. In it, he expounded his astonishingly perceptive theories on disease prevention through healthy living, balancing muscles to prevent injury, and even startling bed designs for spinal alignment. His expositions on wellness, balance, and functional exercise were far ahead of his time and for many decades were only appreciated and experienced by a small number of fortunate people. Ongoing medical research since then has supported a great deal of what he had to say to those that listened. His premise, that functional exercise is the most effective exercise, has continued to develop adherents, and underlies the evolutionary expansion of Pilates' exercises in the 21st Century. Today's awareness and practice can be traced directly back to many of Pilates' very words in *Your Health*.

He was a forward thinking man who based many of his beliefs on the successful past premises in Greek culture. Many fitness gurus, trainers, and training programs continue his work. One can look everywhere at evidence of continuing adaptations and expansions of his fitness regimens and practice. Much of what you can read in Your Health has become incorporated into many different athletic endeavors, healthy living habits and everyday functional skill sets. All of this validates many of his thoughts and beliefs as expressed in the following pages found in his first 1934 publication of *Your Health*.

Pilates used bold phraseology, and colorful imagery, to highlight his physical fitness beliefs. In our adulthood, after years of studying and researching and teaching, we have come to realize the value of Pilates' fitness philosophies. In Chapter 2, misunderstanding "really simple laws of nature" while "searching for normal health and happiness" eventually leads otherwise intelligent men and women to "meander through the valleys of quackery pointing ever downward to suffering, misery and death, instead of climbing to the very pinnacle of the mountain crests of common sense which lead to normal health, happiness and life." Listen to what I am telling you, he says, about natural laws! Read *Your Health* and you will discover for yourself how to address, alleviate and cure many of the "ills of humanity". You will gain the "understanding that really corrects causes rather than merely treats symptoms."

In Chapter 4, Pilates claims that society was racing helter-skelter downward in so far as attaining a balance of mind and body. Not simply wordplay, he believed that civilized society paid more attention to business and mental development at the expense of fitness, health, happiness through natural and normal physical conditioning and activity. Pilates' insight into the causes of unnatural conditions in people led him to many observations about our children. We saw, in the mid Twentieth Century, John F. Kennedy's emphasis on physical fitness and education, decades after Pilates wrote these words. Today, we see a literal explosion of awareness and emphasis on fitness education and practice. Pilates' advice then resonates with the latest educational emphases, both for children and adults:

> My system develops the body and mind simultaneously and nor-
> mally in the home, beginning from infancy and gradually and
> progressively through school and college days to maturity.

In particular, the 21st Century evolution of the Pilates' methods challenges both the brain and the body to learn and to grow.

Ahead of his time, Pilates' Chapter 5 prescription of functional exercise offered common sense remedies for common human ills. In the 21st Century, therapists and medical personnel jointly realize that functional training has direct applicability to activities performed in daily life, with the purposeful goal of performing these daily activities more easily and with less likelihood of injury. The key is to use the mind to control the muscles of the body and to lead them harmoniously to work together effectively.

Chapters 6 and 7 put a name to Pilates' philosophy of fitness --- **Contrology**. He introduces his Greek-based, yet scientific, approach to "supreme physical health, supreme mental happiness and supreme achievements". In the 21st Century, we have seen a wealth of Pilates-inspired practitioners emphasize slow and progressive use of breath work, core muscles, shoulder girdle, and leg/arm control in the many new variations on Pilates exercise themes. The fundamental thread in all of these new developments is the involvement of multiple muscles and joints working together to enhance balance and coordination, endurance and agility, and overall mental and physical strength.

Pilates continues to clarify the aspects of his science of Contrology in Chapter 8, emphasizing the importance and value of forming good habits to children "habits are easily formed - good and bad". His ultimate, and first, lesson is that of correct breathing:

> Children must be taught how to take long, deep breaths,
> sufficient to expand the upper chest to capacity. They must be
> properly instructed how to draw the abdomen in and out at the
> same time holding their breath for a short time. Then they
> should also learn how properly to fully deflate the lungs in
> exhaling.

Researchers in the 21st Century know full well the extraordinary benefits of proper and effective breathing patterns. They also understand much more about the real value of muscle balancing in order to both prevent injuries and rehabilitate athletes (professional and the weekend varieties). Pilates speaks to the "law of natural exercise" in Chapter 8, in which he addresses good posture as well as balance and symmetry in exercise design. This is exactly what has become commonplace in recent exercise research facilities and in the latest certification programs in Pilates' inspired trainings.

Pilates wrote decades ago, and in Chapters 8 and 9, that "the law of natural exercises recognizes "companion" or reciprocal movements in the normal development of the body." He also was very specific in emphasizing the great daily benefits of good posture, and he offered his science of Contrology (now simply Pilates' exercises) as the true answer to the damages wrought by slouching, obesity, and other "violations of the simplest laws of body mechanics."

After decades of experiencing the benefits of Pilates' exercises, understanding his century-old admonitions, and teaching both his original exercises and the 21st Century modifications discussed in this book, we are even more completely in his camp and more firmly impressed with his prescience than ever!

YOUR HEALTH

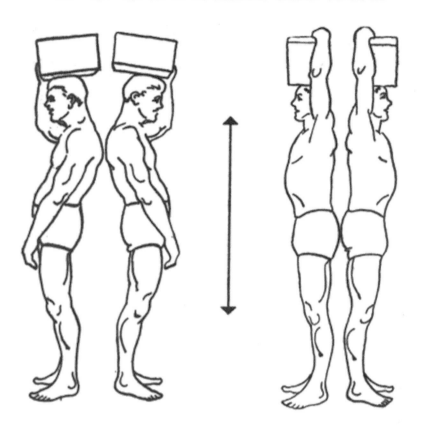

A corrective system of exercising
that revolutionizes the
entire field of physical education.

By Joseph Hubertus Pilates

Your Health – Table of Contents

Chapter 1: A Grave Situation...21

Chapter 2: Health — A Normal-Natural Condition.....................27

Chapter 3: Dreadful Conditions 33

Chapter 4: Heading Downward 38

Chapter 5: Common Sense Remedies for Common Human Ills! 44

Chapter 6: "Contrology" 52

Chapter 7: "Balance of Body and Mind"..................................56

Chapter 8: First Educate the Child! 57

Chapter 9: Proved Facts! 64

Chapter 10: New Style Beds and Chairs..................................71

Your Health

Originally Published in 1934 by Joseph H. Pilates

Prof. Pilates' Health Studios

Where flat feet, curvature of the spine, protruding stomach, stooped-shoulders, hollow chest, hollow back, bow legs, and knocked-kneed conditions are cured through corrective exercises.

Edited, Reformatted and Reprinted
in a New and Easy-to-Read Edition
by Presentation Dynamics

http://www.JosephPilates.org
949-666-5030

Updated with a new introduction by
Judd Robbins and Lin Van Heuit-Robbins
First Published in 1934 by Joseph H. Pilates

Foreword

All new ideas are revolutionary and when the theory responsible for them is proved, through practical application, it requires only time for them to develop and to flourish. Such revolutionary ideas simply cannot be ignored. They cannot be kept in the background.

Time and progress are synonymous terms - nothing can stop either.

Truth will prevail and that is why I know that my teachings will reach the masses and finally be adopted as universal.

Introduction

PERFECT Balance of Body and Mind, is that quality in civilized man, which not only gives him superiority over the savage and animal kingdom, but furnishes him with all the physical and mental powers that are indispensable for attaining the goal of Mankind - HEALTH and HAPPINESS.

The purpose of this booklet is to transmit in a simple form, the causes of present day ill-health and immoral conditions, and the resultant effects which prevent the average human being from attaining this physical perfection - man's inherited birthright.

The author in this booklet tries to teach the reader in simple words the way to correct our present deplorable system of physical and moral education, and to enable each, through a proper understanding of his body, to become fit for the daily tasks ahead of him.

JOSEPH HUBERTUS PILATES

Dedication

I take this means to thank my dear friend, Nat Fleischer, a leading American authority of sports and physical education, for his kind help and suggestions. He has given me added impetus to carry on my work for the betterment of mankind in the construction of corrective apparatus for proper body development. Also my sincere thanks to William J. Miller.

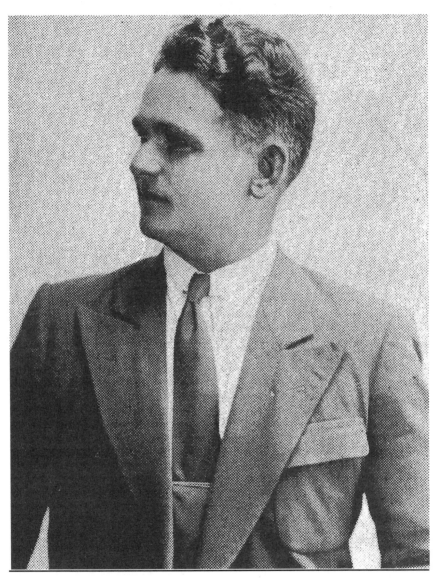

Joseph Hubertus Pilates: *This photograph was taken on his 54th birthday. He has devoted over thirty years to the scientific study, experimentation and research of disturbing troubles which upset Balance of Body and Mind.*

Chapter 1: A Grave Situation

Daily, from sunrise to sunset, the radio, newspapers and magazines broadcast to the world how to maintain health, how to regain health - what to eat, what to drink, and even about what to think.

The conflicting information, expressive of the different opinions of these various health authorities, has proved to be nothing less than "confusion worse confounded" to the millions of radio listeners, readers of newspapers and magazines, who are so unfortunate as to hear or read the diametrically opposed viewpoints of our so-called guardians of our health, since it is rather the exception than the rule, that these instructions are in agreement in their ideas and methods.

To one who has devoted the major portion of his life to the scientific study of the body and practical application of nature's laws of life as pertaining to the natural development of coordinated physical and mental (normal) health and the prevention, rather than the cure of disease, the misinformation he has so often listened to on the air or read, borders closely on the criminal. Why? Because the acceptance of the theories so advanced, not only results in the squandering of untold millions of dollars, but, what is more serious, results in actually shortening, instead of lengthening, the lives of uncounted millions who fall for this bunk.

How many hundreds of thousands die prematurely between the age range of 35 and 59 years, who should rightfully live from 20 to 40 years longer if they but understood and applied the natural laws of life to normal living? Daily we hear the cry for more hospitals, more sanitariums, more homes for the crippled, more lunatic asylums, more reformatories and more prisons!

Who is responsible for this sad, abominable condition? Our so-called health authorities, whose remarks are accepted as law; our so-called scientists, whose statements are religiously accepted - they primarily are to blame because they fail in their mission to civilization!

In the practical universal world, ignorance of the little-understood and much less practiced natural laws of life as applied to normal living is the main cause for the condition referred to. I blame those in control of our health systems for not correcting the evil.

Figures may or may not lie, but the statistics compiled by the United States Army, Navy and Marine Service in the World War, point the way to truth and warn us what health paths to choose and what by-paths to ill-health we should avoid. The record speaks for itself!

How much longer shall this grave situation continue?

Is not this vital question worthy of the closest attention? Should we not have a most vigorous' support of at least a select group of men adequately clothed with the proper official authority and imbued with the necessary inherent idealism to initiate a campaign for the purpose of devoting only a comparatively few hours to an impartial investigation of the merits of my claims herein set forth, even in the face of pessimists' predictions of their failure?

I have proved my case hundreds of times to my pupils and patients, but those who hate to see the old order cast aside refuse to acknowledge the benefits of my system. That's why I've written this book, so that all who are interested may read, digest and know what is wrong with the human race today and how its physical ills can be cured or prevented.

Is it through medicine? No! It is through their efforts, simple exercising, and simple health rules that can and must be observed.

The truth ultimately will burst through the clouds of ignorance and, once in the clear atmosphere, will shine forever in the blue sky of knowledge.

Truth will - must conquer. Instead of pursuing a policy of passivism, aggressive action should and must be taken to bring to light my teachings of health, strength and happiness through proper corrective exercises. The living examples of former broken-down human beings — ill physically and mentally, but now perfect specimens of manhood and womanhood — speaks volumes for my work. Investigate and see for yourself.

It is confidently asserted by me that the statements following, representing my personal views, can be demonstrated and proved:

1 - Barring the writer's own work, there exists today no other fundamental system, no other standard code, designed to gauge, measure and indicate what really constitutes health normalcy. My method, in that respect, is unique and revolutionary. It stands out all by itself.

2 - Not even the medical fraternity as a profession really understands the natural laws of life as applied to normal living, hence the reason for that profession's failure to benefit civilization by proper teaching of health control.

3 - There is today probably not even a single resident professor, scientist or doctor who is really enjoying normal health.

4 - There is today probably not a single private or hospital nurse, or private or professional masseur or masseuse, pseudo or bona-fide physical culture director, who can properly and fully explain what constitutes normal health, and who is a living example of that natural philosophy of health.

5 −In view of the foregoing facts, it is humanly impossible for these uninformed authorities to appreciate at any age the condition, appearance and reactions of the human body in normal health.

6 - The teachers of our children are usually not enjoying ideal health and wholly unable to detect (and therefore unable to correct) the unnatural, harmful habits acquired by their pupils.

7 - Not even the very trainers of our athletes, as well as our outstanding athletes themselves, are with only few exceptions, in any more favorable condition than their fellow creatures, and these often are not even aware of the superior standards of their own condition, which was reached not because of, but in spite of, their lack of information relating to natural methods innocently practiced without their knowledge. They attained their condition rather through the medium of artificial exercises, etc., to which they resorted in striving to realize their ambition to reach the heights of physical perfection, thus resulting in their acquiring more balance of mind and body, than is found in the average person.

8 - Practically all human ailments are directly traceable to wrong habits which can only be corrected through the immediate adoption of right (natural, normal) habits.

9 - The present-day efforts of our so-called health departments are in vain so far as physical health is concerned.

10 - This condition will prevail until such time as marks the recognition of a standard foundation of sound and sane physical culture, based upon the natural laws of life, as applied to the coordination of physical and mental activities tending to the intelligent development of normal health.

11 - All tuberculosis and a veritable legion of other minor ills, not to mention bow-legs, knock-knees, flat feet and curvature of the spine, and heart disease can be prevented (an impossibility under present methods).

12 - The millions of dollars today foolishly expended in the purchase and maintenance of gymnasium equipment, etc., could be more wisely expended for the purpose of training teachers, living examples of normal health, not mere preachers of what normal health (if they really knew) should be.

13 - The millions of dollars today spent on so-called health foods, health talks, and health articles, are actually wasted for the reason that the claims made for them cannot be proved.

14 - Comparatively speaking, only a very small fraction of the money now so spent would, if spent in the right direction, accomplish that most desirable of all aims; namely, restoring the population to normal health, naturally.

15 - Century after century we persisted in sitting and sleeping in unscientifically constructed chairs and beds.

16 - Only today has science discovered that the real cause of our restlessness lies in the fact that our modern chairs, benches and beds are so designed that comfort and relaxation can be had only by constant change of position.

17 - Our chairs, benches, settees, sofas, couches and beds seemingly are designed for every purpose other than that of rest, relaxation or sleep - they are in reality the primary cause of our acquiring wrong and harmful postural habits, too numerous for mention here.

18 - As with chairs and beds, etc., our physical training and sports, with relation to health, are misunderstood.

19 - Only through the attainment of perfect balance of mind and body, can one appreciate what really constitutes normal health.

20 - For over 25 years, the writer has conducted progressive experiments along scientific and practical lines with his own body and those of his pupils, and the complete results of his extensive research along these lines, are now incorporated in the writer's work under his coined name of "Contrology." This represents a brief but comprehensive system of physical culture and is presented in the form of a new art and science, which, if universally adopted and taught in all our educational institutions, will not only tend greatly to eliminate needless human suffering, but will also tend to reduce the necessity for more hospitals, more sanitariums, more homes for the crippled, more lunatic asylums, more reformatories and more prisons. It also will tend to make the expression "health" and "happiness" something more than mere words indicating theoretical conditions rather than the conditions in fact.

Everyone possessing the moral courage owes it to himself and to humanity to investigate the merits claimed for "Contrology" by me.

Chapter 2: Health — A Normal-Natural Condition

Generally speaking, the less the average person merely *talks* about health, the better it is for his health. Not only is health a normal condition, but it is a duty not only to attain but to maintain it. If human beings only knew and only obeyed the simple laws of nature, universal health would follow and the Health Millennium would be here.

Those more or less altruistically engaged in searching for, and studying methods to lessen unnecessary human sufferings, are compelled daily to witness the majority of their fellow-men unknowingly committing grievous sins against Mother Nature. They do this as if their very lives actually depended upon the success of their very efforts, altogether unconscious, however, of the fact that they are really jeopardizing and ruining their future health.

Imagine the immediate good resulting to untold millions, were the energies that are now so wastefully and positively harmfully expended, directed instead into the natural path of least resistance - the road to normal health!

Imagine how many more useful and happy years would be immediately added to their lives!

Imagine how much more they would really enjoy life to its fullest extent!

How many of us, or rather how few of us, realize what Life really is? Unfortunately, this ecstasy of living is reserved for and limited only to those comparatively fortunate few who enjoy normal health - your birthright!

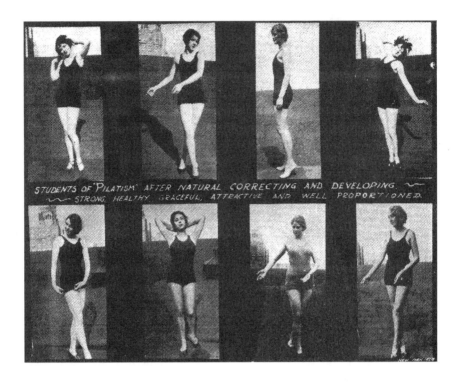

This is a most instructive chart. Here we see some of the girl students who had come to my studio at a time when they were sadly in need of body developing to continue their profession. Each of the persons on this page is a professional singer, actor or dancer. I took them in hand and after three months of my corrective system of exercising, they showed the perfect form and posture seen above. Here we have concrete examples of the benefits derived from my method.

While recognizing that our modern system is to a greater or lesser degree responsible for present health ills, we shall not here attempt to indicate specifically wherein the fault lies. Suffice it to say, that the majority of our so-called intelligent men and women are so utterly and helplessly ignorant of the really simple laws of nature, that in their pitiful searching for normal health and happiness, one invariably finds them needlessly and heedlessly wandering about aimlessly and hopelessly. They meander through the valleys of quackery pointing ever downward to suffering, misery and death, instead of climbing to the very pinnacle of the mountain crests of common sense which lead to normal health, happiness and life.

Were the ailing "traveler" in life not lured by these mirages of false hopes, is it not logical to assume that he would ignore them entirely and courageously about-face and wend his way in the opposite direction? But who is there to warn him against these "mirages" and guide him to the "oasis" of normal health knowledge? These deplorable conditions cannot be attributed either to a want of understanding of natural laws, or their practical and beneficial application to the alleviation and cure of the ills of humanity - an understanding that really corrects causes rather than merely treats symptoms.

Never in history have more "time" and "money" been expended to attain normal physical perfection than in the present era! Never before have vain cravings for normal health been more justified than today!

Great military victories, moral triumphs, scientific achievements and industrial progress are indelibly engraved in the memory of men!

Business men, both during and after the war, were so busily engaged in piling up fortunes that they entirely neglected to devote the necessary time to safeguard their health. Only too late did it finally dawn upon them that in the acquirement of their material fortunes, they, at the same time, carelessly and unthinkingly sacrificed the priceless jewel of their mental happiness, crowned with its physical setting of normal health, which they had so wantonly dissipated. Moreover, they also noted that their relatives and friends, who had followed "The Easiest Way" to fortune so-called, were continually complaining about the state of their poor health.

They saw them pass the remainder of their shortened and spoiled lives, either in constant physical pain or in mental suffering, or both. In many cases they saw them die in the prime of life.

The mistreated body, mindful of its past neglect, eventually exacts its repayment in full with interest in the form of leaving business men their fortunes to contemplate, but denying them the benefits and enjoyments that accrue to other men of wealth blessed with normal health. The bitter lesson has been learned - but too late!

While business men now fully realize that "Everyone Is the Architect of His Own Happiness," they also learn that happiness is primarily dependent upon normal health and not per se upon the mere attainment of social position or monetary wealth. They have learned from practical experience.

Was it not natural to expect that under these inviting circumstances, so-called health specialists, common quacks, proprietors of patent medicines and manufacturers of various forms of mechanical apparatus - lamps, rollers, massaging belts, rowing machines, nostrums, serum and other injections, should, through their advertisements - lure the weaklings? Each quack assures the public that his is the ONLY method of quickly restoring one's health, and he bends his mercenary energies toward reaping the bountiful harvest awaiting him from the lure of the unfortunates, in the form of payments of unwarranted sums for treatments, remedies and services. Such treatments not only fail to accomplish the results desired, but in many cases actually do more harm than good, always, however, the good benefiting only the advertisers at the expense of his innocent victims.

What does this nonsense accomplish? It extracts money from the public without corresponding benefit to the public and for good measure, more often than not, adds to their suffering and misery.

It is very doubtful, indeed, whether a really sane and intelligent person would even think of attempting to prove that any of these many highly recommended "cures" accomplish one iota toward improving the health of anyone, much less effecting a cure.

Pardon this thought - But is it not idiotic, figuratively speaking, to permit one's self to be led around by one's nose by these wholly mercenary, unscrupulous and irresponsible exploiters, who, through their misleading advertisements, fake references and unconscionable methods, prey upon the blind credulity of the public? Think it over, you saps!

Hocus Pocus *is* hocus pocus by any other name!

Under ideal (true) conditions, not only the general public, but physicians as well, will enjoy normal life.

Looking into the future, it is thrilling to those enjoying normal health, in the interest of suffering humanity, to think of the time when through legislative enactment, it will be compulsory for those advocating cures, to demonstrate the efficiency of their methods as reflected in their own physical condition and health.

I stand ready for such test. My method has been proved satisfactory in every detail. My course can stand the acid test before the most critical experts.

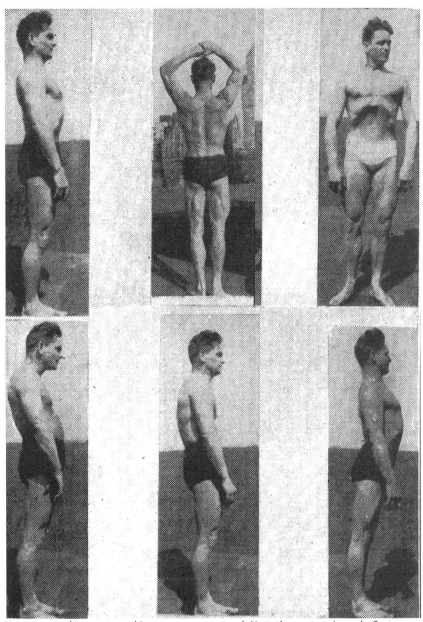

Here we see the correct and incorrect way to stand. Note the posture in each. On top we see three poses, front, side and back. Note the perfect body. Below we have the author posing first, in (A) the Macfadden Hollow Back incorrect posture; (B) the average incorrect posture of an athlete who is broad-shouldered and muscle-bound; (C) the usual position of ninety-five percent of persons, showing protruded stomach (and double curvature of the spine in both lumbar region and the neck.

Chapter 3: Dreadful Conditions

Contrary to the general opinion and popular belief that the mind is absolute master of the body, as expounded by Christian Scientists and others, and contrary to the general opinion and popular belief that the body is absolute master of the mind, as expounded by modern so-called expert physical culture directors and trainers who concentrate their efforts solely on developing the muscles of the body through the medium of various machines and other apparatus, it is contended that neither theory is the correct solution of our centuries-old health problems.

It is contended, however, that the correct solution of our present-day health ills can best be solved only by recognizing the fact that the normal development of the body and mind is possible, not by pitting the body against the mind, or vice versa, which results from concentrating only on the mind or only on the body, as herein indicated, but rather by recognizing the mental functions of the mind and the physical limitations of the body, so that complete coordination between the mind and the body may be achieved.

The theory advocated by this author is safe, sane and sound, whereas the other theories under consideration are more or less unsafe and unsound. That is indicated by the newspapers daily recording the death of some of our most prominent men and women, comprising educators, scientists, inventors, physicians, industrialists, bankers, politicians, actors, lawyers and artists, who, more often than not, die in the very prime of their life. Unfortunately, only too frequently, when they are just reaching the heights of their vocations and when death overtakes them, deprives the world of their most valuable services.

Many of these notables silently suffer untold agonies for years, spurred ever onward by their own ambition to accomplish their aims, and while they themselves and their families are fully cognizant of their condition, the public as a rule, is in entire ignorance of it. These martyrs of false health doctrines die comparatively young, their families are bereaved, their friends are grieved and the world suffers unnecessarily an irreparable loss in their passing.

It is not generally known that many of our most popular misnamed expert physical culture directors and trainers, athletic and other champions, have suffered for years from all various ailments. Especially have they been subject to the dreaded heart disease. In fact, many of these persons die even before they have reached their prime, others right in their prime.

Barring accident, is not this record indicative of the fact that despite their expressed faith in their expounded theories and methods - and one must give them the benefit of the doubt - that they are mistaken in their teachings? Instead of improving their own health and lengthening their lives by the acceptance of practice of their theories and methods, they are, as a matter of fact, actually injuring their health and shortening their own lives, as substantiated by their own untimely death and the record of longevity established by other physical culture authorities, whose theories and methods are diametrically opposed to theirs. The system of the latter must be correct, since the acceptance of practice of their theories and methods by others, as well as themselves, results in improved health and resulting long life - oftentimes exceptionally long life.

Very few of these exponents of physical culture can prove that their doctrines will cause one to live longer and happier than will one who never indulges in any artificial exercise of any kind.

Very few of these so-called physical culturists practice up to 60 or more years what they preach in their youth and very few of them can substantiate their claims as reflected in the condition of their own bodies whenever they do reach those years, if they live that long at all.

It would be exceedingly difficult to find them, for there are not many of them to be found. An impartial investigation would disclose that.

Now is the time for the promotion of a committee composed of influential personages, for the purpose of investigating the sad and deplorable state of ignorance existing with reference to one of the simplest, if not the simplest law of nature - balance of body and mind - and the absence of its practical application in our present-day program of physical education and training.

In these times, with ever-increasing mental training, the human system is more and more dependent on the vitality of the body, which vitality itself is dependent on the absolute coordination of the body and mind - perfect balance!

What is balance of body and mind?

It is the conscious control of all muscular movements of the body. It is the correct utilization and application of the leverage principles afforded by the bones comprising the skeletal framework of the body, a complete knowledge of the mechanism of the body, and a full understanding of the principles of equilibrium and gravity as applied to the movements of the body in motion, at rest and in sleep.

Lacking this knowledge, which is termed "Contrology", physical perfection, with resultant normal life, cannot be attained and comparatively early death cannot be avoided.

Unless the present-day system ignoring the art and science of Contrology are overthrown, it can safely be predicted that they will be successful in accomplishing more harm than good.

On the other hand, if the art and science of Contrology were universally accepted and practiced, one could confidently predict that mental anguish and physical suffering would progressively decrease from generation to generation, and life would be a real pleasure, instead of the curse it now is to so many of our fellow men.

Therefore, it is recommended that the knowledge of the science and art of Contrology should be acquired by all.

Contrology is based upon lessons learned from a life-long study of the principles underlying and governing the laws of nature.

Suffice to say that incorrect habits are responsible for most of our ailments - if not all of them.

Equally true is the statement that only through proper education is it possible to correct bad habits for good ones, the time necessary, depending upon one's condition and age, and while the cost is comparatively nominal, one is assured of regained health arid renewed happiness.

Where can this information be obtained?

Who is qualified to furnish it?

He who criticizes anything without offering something constructive and proved had better not criticize at all.

An idealist and humanist is in duty bound impelled constructively to criticize our present-day systems of physical education and training and prove by actual demonstration in his own body and that of his disciples and students, that they are positively harmful. He must lend his support to effect an immediate change, substituting the correct theory and practice for our current systems.

Accordingly, the undersigned offers - briefly to expound the general principles of his theories and methods covering balance of body and mind, upon which the science and art of Contrology is founded. He offers to demonstrate the truth of his statements to any person desirous of cooperating with him from a more or less altruistic and philanthropic view, in his aim to spread the doctrines of his system and furnish further detailed information regarding his personal ideas on the subject of "tension" and "relaxation," as related to the attainment and maintenance of normal health, so that the world at large may be benefited accordingly.

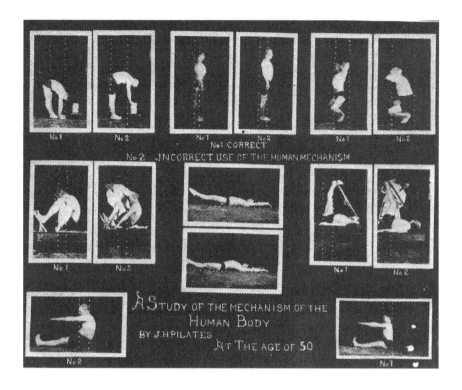

In this plate you see a student and the professor demonstrating the correct and incorrect use of the human mechanism. Study each photograph carefully and see how the body can benefit through my corrective exercises.

Chapter 4: Heading Downward

Are we treading a downward path?

No, we are not "treading" the downward path - rather we are "racing" helter-skelter downward. We are slipping down a path that will lead to the ultimate destruction of the human race, so far as ever realizing the desirable goal of "Balance of Body and Mind" is concerned.

There is only one remedy. The public press must arouse interest to the end that such interest will compel science to "Stop, Look and Listen" at least long enough to permit of an impartial investigation of my claims regarding the simple, sane, safe and sound methods of attaining and maintaining normal health for all. Such an investigation would prove that my teachings will benefit humanity instead of permitting it to be exploited by the unscrupulous.

Science can at one and the same time eliminate poverty, ill health and unhappiness, if it will but investigate *all* and not confine itself only to matters close at hand and make bold to venture far beyond the horizon of its present narrow circle of orthodox activity. I appeal to the intelligent to put an end to the old system and to exploit my scientific system of acquiring and maintaining health.

As civilization advances, we should find the need for prisons, lunatic asylums and hospitals growing steadily less and less. But do we find this to be the case in this era? Certainly not! Teach the human race to care properly for itself and you will do away with these abominable institutions.

What a sad commentary upon our civilization to know that this deplorable "plague" can be annihilated if properly handled, and how criminal it is to think that the "cure" is offered but not accepted because of petty politics and jealousies!

Why boast of this age of science and invention that has produced so many marvelous wonders when, in the final analysis, we find that man has in the race for material progress and perfection, entirely overlooked the most complex and marvelous of all Creations - Man himself!

Were man to devote as much time and energy to himself as he has devoted to that which man has produced, what astounding and almost unbelievable progress would be made; a progress eclipsing all he has so far successfully accomplished, miraculous as that is! Just think that over, my friends.

Man should bear in mind and ponder over the Greek admonition - "Not Too Much, Not Too Little."

Man's neglect of himself, is destructive of his physical and mental efficiency and tends toward the gradual and progressive weakening of his morale with resulting ever-increasing dishonesty, immorality, loss of all true perspective of his responsibilities to himself and to his fellow man, with corresponding loss of idealism and ethical culture. Those are not mere words - they are facts.

Is civilization responsible for man's present-day physical and mental condition? This question is not so difficult to answer if we but try to see with the eyes of the Creator.

Granting that modern science and civilization do not materially benefit the savage from the standpoint of improving his mental capacity, still, at least, he is not harmed or "crippled" from the standpoint of his physical development. This fact can be quickly demonstrated by comparing the physical condition of an average "civilized" man with the physical condition of an average savage.

Logically, man should develop his physical condition simultaneously with the development of his mind - neither should be sacrificed at the expense of the other; otherwise "Balance of Body and Mind" is not attainable, and this very lack of harmony between man's physical and mental health, is primarily responsible for man's unfortunate physical and mental condition today.

If man persists in neglecting himself, or if man continues depending upon effecting cures with present orthodox methods, his case will be increasingly hopeless as time goes on.

Radically different research is necessary in order to discover and apply the laws of nature assuring man of his birthright to "Mental and Physical Balance."

"NOT MIND *OR* BODY BUT MIND *AND* BODY!"

Witness the splendid physique and brute strength of the average savage - his well-proportioned body is the very quintessence of physical beauty - however, brawn has attained the mastery.

Glance at the more or less deformed physique with corresponding lack of strength of the average civilized man. His mal-proportioned body is usually displeasing to the critical eye. However, in his case, the brain has attained the mastery.

What the savage lacks in mental development, the civilized man lacks in physical development. If their physical and mental deficiencies were interchanged without corresponding loss of any of the physical and mental assets each now possess, then the ideal physical condition and mental state would be possible of attainment - "Balance of Body and Mind" would be achieved. What a perfect specimen of human being such an interchange would create!

Relatively speaking, the savage is physically on a par with the beasts, while civilized man is below par, physically, but exceedingly above par, mentally.

Briefly, then, all we need do in traveling the "road of life" is to trace life itself from birth to youth and middle age to discover that which is responsible for disturbing and upsetting physical and mental equilibrium - "Balance of Body and Mind." Then it will be comparatively easy to recognize and understand the causes and to correct them according to the infallible laws of nature. In short, study your body - know its good and bad points - eliminate the bad and improve the good and what will be the result? A perfect man physically and mentally!

Before attempting to modify or reform any established practice or method, we must first know what is wrong before we can even suggest what might be right. Frankly, the indicated truth is that:

The average child is born of parents whose physical and mental balance was either deranged, or, perhaps, never even attained. Often, these parents are physically defective without themselves being aware of the fact, sometimes externally, sometimes internally, and sometimes both.

These physical and organic defects are not without effect upon their children, for they are usually inherited. A high percentage of children are born under unnatural conditions, many others, suffering excruciating pains in the throes of childbirth, and not infrequently sacrificing their lives as well.

Under such unfavorable birth, children are literally born to suffer, and much of the resultant unnecessary suffering is properly charged to the physical condition of the parents. Enumerating a few of the more flagrant faults in man which brings on diseased children, malformation in arms or feet, weak bodies and other things are:

- Feeding children artificial substitutes for mother's milk.

- Feeding children when they are not hungry.

- Overdressing children when they are not cold.

- Forcing children to go to sleep when they are not sleepy.

- Stretching and bending children's arms and legs when they are not inclined to stretch or bend them.

- Compelling children to stand up when they are not strong enough to support their own weight.

- Forcing children to walk when they are not strong enough to control their physical movements.

- Compelling children to sit in chairs for rest (impossible so far as our present-day chairs are concerned), when they are not inclined to do so, preferring rather to "squat" on the floor Turkish-fashion.

- Forcing children to remain physically inactive when they are inclined to be physically active.

- Forbidding older children from climbing trees or jumping fences when their natural inclination is to do so.

- Forcing them to remain quiet when they crave activity. Being compelled to study that which holds no interest for them; they will make the pretense of studying simply to please their "blind" parents.

- Sometimes they are even taught to lie when their natural inclination is to tell the truth.

- Quite commonly, they are deliberately misinformed and taught things they do not understand.

- Children are vaccinated with "poison" to *keep their health.*

- They are forced to swallow laxatives instead of resorting to natural exercise to prevent constipation.

- Children are in these days of prurient prudery, either uninformed or deliberately misinformed regarding sex and permitted to gain such knowledge and information haphazardly in the street and elsewhere to their ultimate ruination in body and mind. Masturbation in both sexes, the curse of mankind, is the result of such handling of children.

- After completing their school day studies, they are compelled to study professions or accept such occupational employment as their parents decide in their "infallible wisdom" is best for them and except in rare cases of rebellion against parental authority, the "victims" resign themselves to their destined fate to the detriment of themselves and society.

- Children are impregnated with the thought that success is measured by the acquisition of money and therefore, their aim should be to become rich as quickly as possible.

- Children are in the same manner forced to go through the routine established for their physical culture education, which system of training is more or less mechanically followed without understanding and under the false impression that this routine is benefiting their health.

Millions upon millions live from the cradle to the grave without really knowing themselves and without really knowing what it is all about. If they are familiar with the Greek adage, "know thyself", it is not practically applied to themselves. These children in adolescent and adult life, lacking normal initiative, appetites, passions and the stress of competition, figuratively speaking, slowly sink to a low level, never experiencing the thrills of life, never experiencing the glory of successful accomplishment, and never enjoying the fruits of over-flowing vitality and health that should be theirs if taught the problems of life and the proper control of the body.

Later on, when their vitality is at low ebb, they begin to shrivel at their extremities, their blood pressure is either subnormal or abnormal - their heads get too warm, their feet and hands get too cold - their mentality waxes and wanes and they are, so to speak, more or less animated "clothes racks." This is a mighty serious problem. Think it over. It is deserving of every person's consideration.

And then again, they are influenced to join athletic teams, docilely submitting to a more or less brutalizing training regime, usually concentrating all their efforts on the physical development of the body and the acquirement of physical strength without any regard whatsoever to the acquisition and development of mental control. They are drilled to do stunts for which their bodies are unfit. While their bodies are either underdeveloped or overdeveloped, their mental control is absolutely neglected.

Is this the kind of instruction you want your children to have? Wouldn't the human race be better off if such system were abolished?

Do not all these violations of the simple laws of nature lead us to tread the downward path? I offer the human race in the place of the present orthodox methods, something revolutionary in character and results, "BALANCE OF BODY AND MIND" through the study and practice of the science of 'CONTROLOGY." My system develops the body and mind simultaneously and normally in the home, beginning from infancy and gradually and progressively through school and college days to maturity.

But will those behind the orthodox system of ruination, accept my new, revolutionary system of training? Not until public opinion forces them to do so, for they well realize that once my system is accepted generally, which must be the case soon, it will mean the end of the quacks, the crooks who wouldn't dare to undergo the very training they offer you as a build-up process to health.

Chapter 5: Common Sense Remedies
for Common Human Ills!

Whether or not we are conscious of it, it is nevertheless a fact, that in the course of our daily activities, if we live a normal life, we receive the benefit of natural exercises - those performed in every movement we make. These very necessary functional activities, experienced by one living a normal life, preclude all necessity for undertaking artificial exercise of any kind.

It is really a rank falsity to believe that one cannot be both strong and healthy without having first to indulge in more or less violent training "stunts," but unfortunately this erroneous concept is so firmly entrenched in the minds of the general public, that it would probably require the omnipotent power of a deity to dispel this universally accepted nonsense from their minds.

However, in order that one may receive the maximum benefit and resulting normal health from one's daily activities, one should understand at least some of the more rudimentary underlying principles governing the mechanism of the human body in motion, rest and sleep. For example, the leverage possibilities of the bones composing its skeletal framework, the range and limitation of proper muscle tension and relaxation, the laws of equilibrium and gravity, and last but not least, how to inhale and exhale; i.e., how to breathe properly - normally. Knowledge of these is essential if we are to benefit from any exercises.

Since the public seemingly is either uninformed or misinformed with reference to these principles, they cannot of necessity benefit by them, which fact is only too self-evident when one, who is himself thoroughly versed in the knowledge of physical education, measures humanity in terms of normal health. If this knowledge were universally disseminated and the system advocated for its propagation, universally adopted both laymen and professionals, as well as by the properly constituted health authorities in particular, what a splendid human race we would see.

Again, the simple truth is repeated, that one may both attain and maintain perfect (normal) health without resorting to the expedient of artificially exercising the body. This statement seems to be fully substantiated when one observes the perfection of physical form, strength, grace, agility, endurance, health and longevity in the animal kingdom. With man it is just to the contrary.

Has the natural exercise instinctively indulged in by such "life" anything to do with the uniform attainment and maintenance of their ideal physical condition, as reflected in their natural beauty and normal health? Has the indulgence of artificial exercise advocated by man for man, anything to do with the uniform failure of his attainment to even reach much less maintain a similar degree of ideal physical condition, as is reflected in his natural beauty and normal health?

Would animal life benefit by exchanging instinct for man's ability to think? Or, would man benefit by exchanging ability to think for the animal's instinct?

Judging from an impartial study of their respective physical conditions, one must admit that were animals and men respectively to interchange their instinct and ability to think, that the animals would have bargained their birthright away for a "mess of pottage," while man would have gained immeasurably by the exchange, at least to the extent of physical perfection.

Did you ever hear of an animal gymnasium conducted by animals for animals, for the purpose of gratifying their desire or need for artificial exercising?

Is it not true that animals in their natural state and in their natural habitat exercise naturally as a matter of course?

Do animals understand natural laws and govern themselves accordingly? The answer is "yes" because instinct unerringly guides all living creatures including man himself.

Have you ever closely and thoughtfully observed the movements of a newly-born babe? If you have studied animal life at all, you will have been impressed by the fact that so far as physical actions and movements are concerned, animals are men and men are animals. You see that in the movements of a new-born baby.

Both animals and men move their bodies in all possible directions; freedom of bodily action is paramount. This constant desire for change in movement in babies is only a manifestation of one of the many fundamental laws of nature - the law of action - which animals and human beings obey alike, if unhampered.

Natural instinct prompts mothers of the animal kingdom to permit nature to "take its course" as long as the lives of their offspring are not in danger. However, if one of the members of their sometimes rather large families seems to be inclined to laziness and disinclined to "play," its mother will not hesitate to force it to move about so that its muscles may be properly developed and strengthened through increased circulation of the blood. She will go even to the extent of grasping the "culprit" by its neck in her mouth and shaking and dropping it repeatedly on the ground until the lazy one responds to the hint. Have you ever watched a cat and her kittens or a dog and its litter?

How differently does the human mother act!

Instead of permitting infants and growing children the opportunity freely to obey their natural "instinct," as evidenced by their desire for action - constantly turning around, grasping for and holding on to objects within their reach, stretching and bending their little bodies, arms and legs; creeping on the floor and playing in the sand or on the grass until their little muscles tire naturally, and then fall into a healthy sleep as intended by another law of nature, the fond mothers literally stuff their offspring's' stomachs with food to overflowing capacity, and then "pack" their tender bodies in bandages after first (wholly unintentionally and solely through ignorance or misinformation on the subject) cruelly locking the joints of their hips and knees.

In order to pacify their resulting crying protests against this rather inhuman treatment, the mother next proceeds to rock the child to sleep. Is it a natural sleep they thus get? No, the little innocents are either nauseated or half unconscious or both when they finally fall asleep from mere exhaustion.

How differently acts the dumb animal mother from the human mother!

The animal mother feeds her young ones as indicated by her instinct. Then she permits them to fall asleep, allowing them to assume their natural positions usually against her own warm body, which not only afford the little ones the necessary bodily resistance required for their complete comfort, but also gives them the benefit of the healthful magnetism of the mother's own body, an essential and vitally important factor in the welfare and well being of her offspring.

No college education is needed to understand what these remarks are meant to convey; namely, to observe what the "seeing" eyes see and to use common sense in the bringing up of our children. If only a very small fraction of the time and money now spent on research work were spent in the study of the many violations of the laws of nature for educational purposes, how much more would life be enjoyed and appreciated than it is possible to enjoy and appreciate life at the present time?

One understanding the subject-matter of this discussion may be pardoned for taking the liberty of discussing matters which are usually discussed only by scientists and doctors with degrees. Every free-born man endowed with common sense blessed with idealism, and prompted by humanitarian motives, instinctively feels it to be his duty to "cast his bread" (his own knowledge) "upon the waters" so that his brethren who may still believe in the observance of the ethical laws governing human intercourse, may benefit thereby.

Everyone is invited - no one is barred - to follow those in search of right and wrong and form his own opinion accordingly. In this instance, one begins his journey for knowledge, tracing it from boyhood to middle and old age, with the idea of testing the truth of these statements.

The child we left innocently sleeping in its cradle is now wide awake and lying on its little back, but, believe it or not, without the barbarous bandages, and with its hunger already satisfactorily appeased, it is enjoying the liberty of complete freedom in legs, arms and body improvements.

Isn't it strange that now, for some reason or other, we feel the same child unhampered by the bandages previously applied to securely lock its hips and knees when it was first put to sleep?

Most people seem to think that bandaging the lock hips and knees of sleeping and resting children is absolutely necessary in order that the legs may grow straight. What folly!

One never heard of animals resorting to this or similar artificial means for stretching the legs of their growing young and neither do we find savages resorting to such devices. Furthermore, since barring accident, we find the average savage and the average animal in nature in normal physical condition, blessed with well-proportioned bodies, and bow-legs, knock-knees, and double curvature of the spine conspicuous by their absence, we must reach the logical conclusion that the deformities children ordinarily suffer have been brought on by the terrible treatment they received as a baby.

If the reader has the ambition and patience to follow this discussion to its eventual conclusion, he might ultimately be convinced that adherence to this time-worn tradition of bandaging the child's body is really one of the first of the many bad habits which ignorant parents force upon their helpless children, a condition for which the health authorities are responsible.

The average normal unhampered child in attempting to gratify its perfectly natural desire for muscular movement will naturally assume the so-called "spread-eagle" position, constantly stretching and bending its arms and legs, lifting its head up and down, and turning from left to right and vice versa. If left undisturbed, it manifests supreme contentment and keen joy, but after a more or less prolonged period of this state, it will begin to manifest evidence of uneasiness and unhappiness which condition if unrelieved, will bring on a crying spell. Then, if the cries are unheeded, the child will become exhausted, unless the parents intercede and change it to another position which the child is not strong enough to assume by itself.

Practically nine out of every ten mothers will confidently tell you that the reason the child cried was because it wanted to be carried in the arms, and this explanation seemingly is partly true, at least, because the child immediately ceases crying when its tiny legs are resting against its mother's body.

However, that is but another popular fallacy that needs to be exploded.

Why does the child really cry?

The correct answer to this question is quickly and definitely ascertainable. All that is necessary is for the experimenter to lie on his back in the same position as that assumed by the child and make the same movements for a period ranging from only 20 to 40 minutes, whereupon he will know what happens and then he will know why the child is restless and cries.

As it is, no one really seems to know what happens; otherwise, this cruelty would have been abandoned long ago.

However, if the child were lying in a normal bed – one designed in conformance with the fundamental principles underlying and governing the anatomical balance of its bony structure - it could lie for hours at a time in any given position without experiencing any undue strain. Lacking the advantage inherent in such a scientifically designed and constructed bed, its position must, of necessity, from time to time, be changed, first from one position, then to another, so that if the child is found crying while resting on its back, the crying will immediately cease if it is turned to rest on its stomach and vice versa.

This change of position is now absolutely necessary for the child's comfort and if these changes be made at more or less frequent intervals, they will materially assist the child in the performance of its natural exercise, so essential and vitally important to its proper development. This procedure makes for the child's contentment and happiness and permits it to grow up strong and healthy.

Another form of mistreatment of young children is that of forcing them to sit quietly in a chair in a right angle (upright) position. What it really means to sit quietly in our modern dining room, kitchen and other chairs, for even only a comparatively short period of time, is something that those conducting our research laboratories have evidently failed to personally ascertain, for if they had, they certainly would have relegated the present type of chairs to limbo centuries ago and advocated the construction of the chairs which I have invented and recommend.

I challenge any person to sit quietly, free from all movements, for one hour in any modern chair. You'll soon learn what it means to the child. The muscles have become so cramped and numbed, that they are no longer sensitive to feeling. No one could really rest in such a position, because the position itself is a most unnatural one. For the naturally correct position, assuring the maximum amount of rest and comfort, it is suggested that one look around and watch the position that children naturally assume when they are left alone.

Does one naturally assume uncomfortable positions? Assuredly not. Then why not permit the child to "squat" on the floor, Turkish-fashion, American-Indian, Japanese and savage fashion, which position is at one and the same time natural, comfortable and healthful.

Children at this young age prefer and enjoy sitting on the floor, moving around bear-fashion on "all-fours" or creeping on their hands and knees, all of which develop the larger muscles of their backs, legs, stomach and shoulders.

Proud (and unintentionally cruel) parents, seriously interfere with and disrupt this natural course of bodily development by forcing the children to start walking or standing upright before their muscles have been sufficiently developed properly to support their weight and before they have the mental capacity to control their equilibrium in movement. Normal children require no parental instruction or help in this direction, for the simple reason that if they are left to themselves, they will naturally keep on learning and trying until they are able, not only to stand in an upright position without falling, but also until they have acquired the ability to walk by themselves.

To force children to follow any other procedure than this natural one, no matter how well-intentioned, is detrimental to the best interests of their health. Curvature of the spine, bow-legs, knock-knees, faulty posture and later on flat feet, are directly traceable to these mistaken ideas. They have their origin in the deplorable ignorance of their fond but ignorant parents.

How much more common sense or natural instincts have dumb animals?

How entirely different is their method of "bringing up" their young ones?

How much fun can we have simply by watching the animal mother especially of the cat family, giving a lesson in physical culture to her offspring?

What a lesson she can teach us!

Chapter 6: "Contrology"

The ancient Greeks probably knew better than anyone else, the true meaning of "Balance of Body and Mind," as tangibly expressed in terms of supreme physical health, supreme mental happiness and supreme achievements along the highway of human progress. They even believed that the soul itself is inextricably bound up with the physical functions and mental manifestations of the human body.

They fully understood that the nearer one's physique approached the state of physical perfection, the nearer one's mind approached the state of mental perfection.

They knew that the simultaneous and co-equal development of one's ability voluntarily to control one's body and mind was a paramount law of nature and that the unequal (abnormal or subnormal) development of either the body or the mind, or the neglect of either or both, would result in the complete failure to realize the very first law of civilization - (preservation of life) - the attainment and maintenance of one's bodily and mental perfection. Failing realization of this desirable aim, the body would become, as it were, an "'enemy" of the mind and vice versa, whereas the mind should become as it were, a "friend" of the body and vice versa.

Unlike so many of our fellowmen of today, the Greeks religiously practiced what they preached, as witness the marvelous state of their achieved physical perfection as reflected in their wonderful statues.

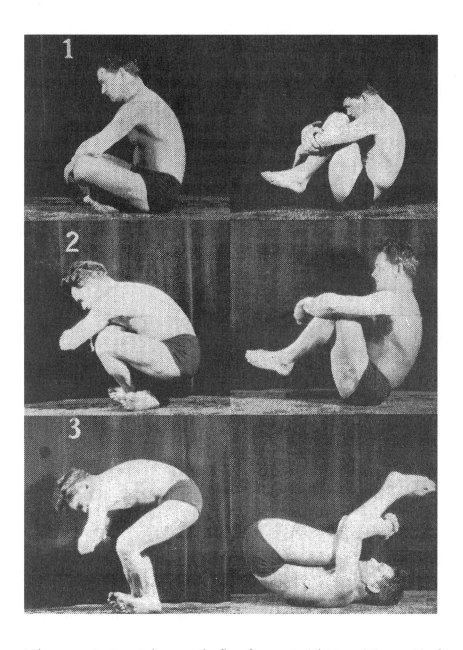

Did you ever try to get down on the floor from a straight to a sitting position? Try it. Having trouble? Of course you are, because there is a lack of coordination. Note the pictures on this page showing through Contrology the grace with which this can be done. Note the perfect curve, elasticity, and flexibility of the spine - the perfect mechanism of hip, knee and ankle joints.

In view of their unique physical and mental development, is it not logical that they should have established themselves as outstanding intellectuals and have been numbered among the "spokes" if they did not really constitute the very "hub" of the "wheel" of civilization?

Unfortunately for us all, their striking lesson seems to have been absolutely lost to modern civilization. What a pity!

With all our progress in many other directions, we still, so far as the harmonious and scientific development of our bodies and minds is concerned, have actually retrograded from their high standards of co-equal development of body and mind. Comparatively speaking, we are today really living in the "jungles of ill health and unhappiness", whereas the ancient days, man was living on the very "mountain tops of actual health and happiness".

The athletic prowess of the Greeks was continually being publicly demonstrated in their splendid and commodious athletic arenas, so that the masses could note the perfect bodies and seek to emulate the athletes.

Their beautifully developed and well-proportioned bodies proved an inspiration to sculptors, who immediately recognized the "living art" before their very eyes and perpetuated it in the unsurpassed marble classical Grecian statues now exhibited in our various world-renowned museums. That is one of the richest of legacies left to us by ancient Grecian civilization.

Truly are they an object lesson to us moderns that we should not overlook. Particularly should our duly constituted health authorities give heed to this lesson in health culture through recognition and practice of the fundamental principles governing "Balance of Body and Mind" in the attainment and maintenance of physical and mental perfection as the Greeks did.

The mode of living prevalent amongst the ancient Greeks was, of course, entirely different from that of today. These people were nature-lovers. They preferred to commune with the very elements of nature itself - the woods, the streams, the rivers, the winds and the sea. All these were natural music, poems and dramas to these Greeks who were so fond of outdoor life.

Their bodies were not unnecessarily burdened with clothing, as we understand it today. They preferred to more or less expose their bodies to the invigorating air and revitalizing rays of the sun, all of which, of course, made it possible for them to achieve their goal of physical and mental perfection to a greater degree than is possible today.

Were our athletes today to pursue the system advocated and practiced by these ancient Greeks, it is confidently predicted that with our present knowledge of "Contrology," they would not only reach the same high standard of physical and mental perfection achieved by the Grecians in their day, but as a matter of fact (incredible as it may seem), would actually surpass it, particularly when we view human nature "en masse" and compare it with the "en masse" standards established in ancient Greece.

The Greeks did not as fully understand the laws governing "Balance of Body and Mind" as it is understood by us today. Were we to discontinue much of our present mode of living and discard our present systems of physical training, and instead, adopt such training as I here advocate, based upon the science of "Contrology," there would result a rejuvenation of mind and body and living itself would again become an art as it was in the days of the ancient Grecians.

Habits of nature, rather than artificial training and exercises, would maintain one in perfect physical and mental condition.

Immediately following, I will explain in brief the general principles underlying "Balance of Body and Mind" - a science to which I have devoted many years' study.

Chapter 7: "Balance of Body and Mind"

A sound mind "housed" in an unsound body (50% balance) is just about as desirable a physical condition as is the structural weakness of a house boasting a fine copper roof but built upon a foundation of shifting sand.

A sound body "housing" an unsound mind *(50%* balance) is just about as desirable a physical condition as is the structural weakness of a house boasting a solid rock foundation but possessing a roof of flimsy paper.

A sound mind "housed" in a sound body (100% balance) is desirable just as is a fine copper-roofed house built on a solid rock foundation.

An unsound mind "housed" in an unsound body (no balance) is undesirable just as is a flimsy-papered roof house built on a shifting sand foundation.

What do the foregoing statements with their accompanying figures indicate?

Obviously, they clearly indicate that neither the mind nor the body is supreme - that one cannot be subordinated to the other.

Both must be coordinated, in order not only to accomplish the maximum results with the minimum expenditure of mental and physical energy, but also to live as long as possible in normal health and enjoy the benefits of a useful and happy life.

Chapter 8: First Educate the Child!

In childhood, habits are easily formed - good and bad. Why not then concentrate on the formation of only good habits and thus avoid the necessity later on in life of attempting to correct bad habits and substituting for them good habits - oftentimes impossible even when the physical exertion is accompanied by equally strenuous mental efforts.

Therefore, it is of paramount importance that the child be taught the major principles of "Balance of Body and Mind." In other words, the proper development of body and mind, through the new science of "Contrology," is what must he taught the child.

Generally speaking, physical culture methods employed in our schools today may appeal to the uninformed laymen, but to one who has a knowledge of the subject, as I have, they would be amusing were it not for the fact that they are deplorable in their efforts.

In classroom and gymnasium alike (invariably either overcrowded or inadequately ventilated or both), we see children exercising a few minutes daily as a matter of routine.

Few children understand the significance of these insignificant movements of their arms, legs and body, and only a very few exercise with vigor.

The great majority mechanically exercise without mental concentration - an utter waste of time and effort. Such exercising leads to false conceptions and conclusions in adult life highly detrimental to the ultimate welfare of the grown-up child.

Before any real benefit can be derived from physical exercises, one must first learn how to breathe properly - this all-important function requires individual instruction, not only by precept but by example.

It is wholly insufficient to tell the individual to inhale and to exhale. To learn to breathe properly is really more difficult an accomplishment than the average (uninformed) person realizes. Moreover, there are comparatively few teachers who understand the art of correct breathing and who are capable of instructing others in the art.

"Carriage of the Body" is freely preached, but what the correct carriage of the body is, is not understood.

One constantly hears the expressions "heads up" and "shoulders back." In the effort to throw the shoulders back, the individual hollows his back too much (bow-like) and forces his shoulder blades against his spine, and most harmful of all protrudes his stomach.

That the instructions themselves are unnatural and without benefit, is of secondary importance to the fact that they are dangerous to one's health, which is of primary importance.

What really is desired is not the backward throw of the shoulders as previously indicated, but rather the simultaneous drawing in of the stomach and the throwing out of the chest.

The average child (uninformed) when standing, hands in pocket, abdomen protruding, shoulders stooped forward, legs too far back, joints locked and feet at the wrong angle, is not being benefited by this condition as all of these postures, of course, are not conducive to forming good habits but are responsible for bow-legs, knock-knees and later on, flat feet.

Were the child in the first instance, taught the difference between right and wrong, he would naturally avoid what is wrong and follow what is right. Particularly in the matter of breathing, this early instruction is of vital importance.

In their normal (natural) condition, children do not need the stimulus of artificial exercise. Unfortunately, however, children born to live under the influence of the artificialities, require a special course in mind training in order that they may consciously control their bodily movements until the good habits formed become subconscious routine acts.

The first lesson is that of correct breathing.

Children must be taught how to take long, deep breaths, sufficient to expand the upper chest to capacity. They must be properly instructed how to draw the abdomen in and out at the same time holding their breath for a short time. Then they should also learn how properly to fully deflate the lungs in exhaling.

To properly deflate the lungs is an art in itself and this final step in correct breathing is least understood. As a rule, it is seldom, if ever, properly taught unless the individual is privately coached by one who understands what it really is all about.

Correct breathing exercises under the dominance of mental control, would undoubtedly accomplish more toward the prevention of tuberculosis as well as accomplish more toward attaining and maintaining maximum health standards, than all other remedies combined.

The lungs cannot be completely deflated at first without considerable effort. With perseverance, however, the desired results can be accomplished and with increasing power, gradually and progressively develop the lungs to their maximum capacity. That will actually cause the chest to "balloon" and at the same time bring practically every other muscle of the entire system into play. Thus the child's posture will then be normal (natural).

With proper breathing and correct posture, the child has no need for artificial exercise. Walking, running, jumping, tumbling, climbing, wrestling, etc., are natural exercises calculated by Mother Nature to develop her children normally.

The law of natural exercise precludes the hobby idea altogether in the matter of exercise, unless one is really and seriously desirous of not seeking symmetrical development of one's body.

For instance, the left side of the body must not be developed while the right side of the body is wholly neglected.

The law of natural exercises recognizes "companion" or reciprocal movements in the normal development of the body.

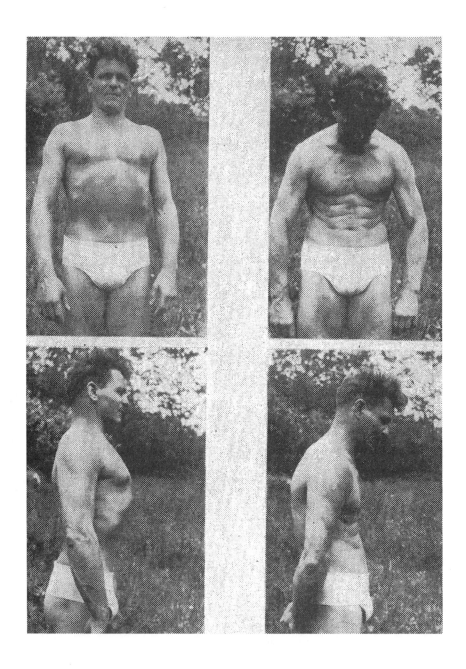

Here we have four photographs showing the correct way to breathe - two side poses and two front views of natural breathing. Note in each the chest at the point of inhaling and when exhaling. The first is the inhale movement, the second, the exhale movement.

For example, if a series of natural movements call for a definite number of forward bends, then this series should be repeated by a definite number of backward bends and so on, ad libitum.

"Hardening" of the body is another most important consideration in the matter of its proper and normal (natural) development.

Correct clothing plays a leading role in this regard. Children, if left to follow their own natural inclinations, without restraint, will not hesitate to discard unnecessary garments. In fact, the fewer the clothes, the better they like it.

The more active one is in outdoor physical recreation activities, the less need there is for unnecessary clothing. Children seldom, if ever, contract colds under such circumstances, but the moment these activities cease, nature prompts them to seek the necessary clothing protection to avoid chills.

Children should be permitted to exercise in the open air irrespective of normal weather conditions, barring storms and severely cold spells, because the open air is Nature's tonic that strengthens their bodies naturally and "hardens" them accordingly.

If the child comes home from play complaining of feeling a chill, or cold, it should be given a good hot and cold shower and, after a little rest, sent out again to rejoin its playmates so that its body may gradually and progressively become accustomed to its natural regime.

Many are the sins committed by uninformed persons in following false theories and methods for accomplishing this highly desirable result. The more natural and simple the method, the better.

Experience has taught us that it is the part of wisdom to practice very early in life exposing the young child's nude body to the air and sun as much as possible. No restrictions should be placed upon natural exercises so long as their indulgence does not indicate danger to health and life.

Much of the child's welfare depends upon cleanliness of the skin. Water should be freely used. Hot shower baths followed by gradually cooler and cooler temperature until the water is cold, has a most beneficial and exhilarating effect, especially when the body is briskly "massaged" (at the beginning) with a soft brush to be later on discarded for a harder one.

Soap should be used only occasionally as when the body is covered with perspiration. In all other instances, the brush massaging answers the purpose. This system of skin treatment not only is responsible for its soft texture and pink glow, but by removing all the soap residue lodged in the pores of the skin, opens these pores, thus permitting them to function naturally and eliminating the cause of colds.

Children should also be taught when washing or taking a tub or shower bath, to cup some water in the hollow of one hand and while holding one nostril closed, with the other hand, snuff this water up in the other free nostril, expel it by pressing both nostrils slightly, and repeat for the other nostril.

In this connection, if the water is permitted to enter the throat and ejected through the mouth, the throat and mouth are cleansed and kept in a healthy condition and gradually immunized against disease. These simple suggestions, if properly followed, would prevent the majority, if not all of our nose, mouth and ear ailments.

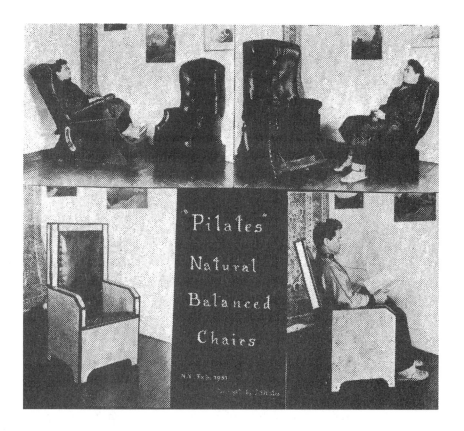

The above plate shows some of the many models developed by the author to insure correct posture and to rest the body perfectly. There is a chair for every purpose - from the kindergarten child to the aged adult suffering from the physical ailments so prevalent in old or middle age from the effects of bad posture and lack of exercises.

Chapter 9: Proved Facts!

Practically everyone knows that nature has endowed human beings, and certain animals, with a "backbone," but few recognize that state of perfection which nature intends the human spine to reach through the medium of its scientific, progressive, and natural development from birth to maturity, so that the "ridge-pole" of the human "house" may properly grow into normal form (straight). Still less understand the mechanism of the spine and the proper methods of training this "foundation" bone of the body so that its movements will be under their absolute control at all times. Most persons are not aware of the fact that, by reason of this utter lack of understanding, the human spine has been sadly neglected, for many, many generations.

Accordingly, it has been permitted to develop itself, as it were, to fit the individual cases, with the result that the average human spine today invariably is more or less deformed. The prevalence of this condition, unfortunately, has been too generally accepted by the public as normal. Some of our leading anatomists, likewise, seemingly, hold similar beliefs. This state of affairs is truly deplorable since it not only gives credence to a grievous error, which, if not immediately corrected, will continue to bar the victims of this gross misunderstanding from traveling the road to ultimate recovery, and prevents them from reaching their goal of normal health.

At no time in the history of medicine was it more important than it is right now, that organized science undertakes an impartial investigation of the facts herein presented and supplements them by an intensive study of this all-important subject.

In view of the revolutionary inventions and the never-ceasing research in laboratory and afield, medical science should be emboldened to discard its old-fashioned ideas as well as its orthodox methods of instruction, and concentrate upon ways and means of preventing rather than curing disease. That is why I am preaching the sermon embodied in this book.

Consideration and examination of proved facts pertinent to this subject should quickly convince unbiased medical and other authorities that the human body has for centuries been tortured unnecessarily by reason of our failure to recognize and understand the underlying principles governing the natural mechanism of the human spine, as well as recognizing and understanding the factor of equilibrium with reference to its application to the human body - in motion, at rest, and at sleep. That is a study I have made and upon that study I have invented chairs, mattresses and beds for the proper development of the spine.

It is the duty of the humanist to direct attention to this important matter, based upon observation and experience rather than to enter into merely controversial arguments with anatomists regarding divergent views on this subject.

Without undue reiteration (reference to standard medical literature is readily accessible) to the subject of these remarks - "the anatomy of the human spine" - the following is presented:

1 - Knowledge based upon fact regarding the mechanism of the human spine is woefully insufficient. This deplorable lack of knowledge is primarily responsible for the present-day acceptance of abnormal and subnormal conditions as normal, which in turn is responsible for practically every ailment afflicting mankind today.

2 - Spine curves as depicted by anatomists represent on the average the actual conditions usually found in the human body, but instead of being accepted as normal, should be rightfully considered either abnormal or subnormal as the case may be.

Practically 95 per cent out of every one hundred persons examined are afflicted with an abnormal spine curvature. See photograph No. 1.

Undoubtedly, it is this very "preponderance of evidence," the 95 percent of malformation of spines, which leads anatomists and others to the false conclusion that since so many have this curvature, that represents the ideal and thus the normal condition of the human spine.

Furthermore, it is contended that this curving of the spine is necessary not only to lend added strength to the spine itself, but also that it may better absorb vibrations to which it is constantly subjected.

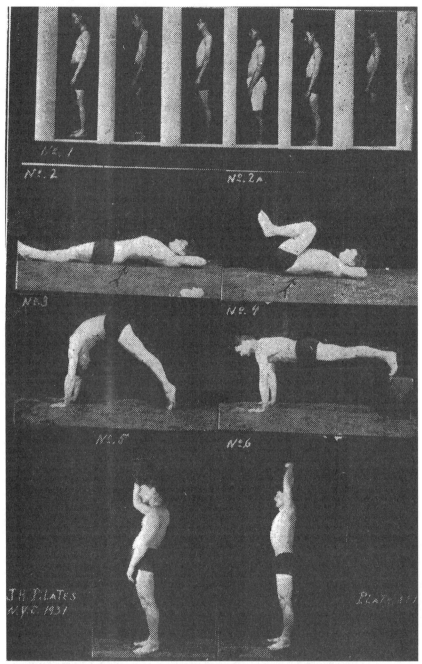

Photographs 1-6: Here is a chart giving proved facts regarding the curvature of the spine. It shows that the spine must be straight.

Has not science grievously erred in this instance in view of the fact that its unqualified acceptance of this conclusion is in violation of the simplest law of body mechanics?

3 - The spine of every normal child is straight. The back is perfectly flat.

Fortunately for its own benefit, the growing child inherits sonic natural movements such as that of bending the knees and assuming the natural curled position in sleep. Thus the child-animal (pardon the expression), subconsciously seeks the most comfortable natural position affording its bones just the right degree of resistance to achieve this desirable result.

It is almost criminal, to insist upon the child lying flat with legs outstretched and joints "locked" in a bed equipped with our more or less elastic modern bedsprings as most parents do.

Forcing the child to assume these unnatural positions incidentally reacts upon several groups of muscles, especially the major muscles, which is reflected in their tensed or semi-tensed condition, according to the extent of the child's deviation from the normal-natural positions.

Naturally, this unnatural posture is both uncomfortable and more or less painful, as evidenced by crying until the vicious habit of wrong position is more or less permanently formed. Later on, the child perpetuates this harmful custom when parenthood blesses it with children and so on.

How much physical damage and suffering are due to this unpardonable mistake?

Photograph #2 admirably illustrates the bad effects caused by this practice of unduly taxing the muscles by the resultant steady straining pull unnecessarily inflicted upon them and which constant pull tends to draw the spine out of a straight line - its normal position. As the child grows older and reaches the walking stage, its spine assumes a more or less pronounced curve, particularly if parents, through neglect or ignorance, permit the child to slouch, and deny it the benefit of natural exercise, such as creeping and tumbling on the ground. These parental prohibitions detrimentally affect their off-spring's development and jeopardize their attaining normal health.

Not satisfied with this inhibition, the "head of the family" and his "better half" make matters even worse by insisting that the child stand on its legs before the muscles in the upper portion of his legs and the muscles of its back are sufficiently developed to support its weight.

These muscles are developed naturally and normally by permitting the child to run on "all fours" bear fashion, or at least by allowing it to creep on its hands and knees and after many trials with accompanying falls, to stand up leaning against the wall, chairs, beds, etc.

Every normal child, if left alone, will quite naturally and without parental help, try and try and try to move about from point to point as herein previously indicated. Knowingly to force the child to stand on its weak and undeveloped legs, is positively cruel.

The penalties are resultant curvature of the spine - are bow-legs, knock-knees and later on in life, so-called flat feet. The suggestion advanced that the curve in the spine affords additional strength to the vertebrae column, is scarcely borne out by even a cursory study of simple mechanical principles.

Photographs 3 and 4 furnish convincing proof that a lateral arch is undeniably stronger than a horizontal plane, while photographs 5 and 6 aptly demonstrate the fact that a curved line up right is not as strong as a straight line.

Therefore, is it not logical to conclude from the foregoing illustrations and observations, that there is no justification for accepting the curved spine as indicative of normal? Rather is it not conclusive evidence that just the contrary is the truth?

Accordingly, by the same token, should not remedial steps be taken forthwith to correct the disadvantages arising from the continued acceptance of this false philosophy regarding the human spine?

The photographs submitted tell the story even better than the writer's words can do, since they are life examples and appeal to the eye as well as to the mind.

For instance, photograph 6 illustrates perfectly and furnishes adequate justification for the writer's conclusion that the normal spine should be straight to successfully function according to the laws of nature in general and the law of gravity, in particular. Photograph 5, aside from being unaesthetic, illustrates only too tragically the ills inherent in the backward curve - decreasing force bordering close to no force whatsoever, mere feebleness, "dis-grace," the curve itself being especially dangerous to the vital organs and the body in general.

The slouch position illustrated in the foregoing paragraph (the pelvis is pressed forward), upsets the equilibrium of the body resulting in disarrangement of the various organs affected including the bones and muscles of the body as well as the nerves and blood vessels, not overlooking the glands. More or less permanently harmful injuries sustained, are not recorded here.

5 - Abdominal obesity and the dangerous effects of corpulence have their origin in the "mis-carriage" of the spine.

Proper carriage of the spine is the only natural preventive against abdominal obesity, shortness of breath, asthma, high and low blood pressure and various forms of heart disease. It is safe to say that none of the ailments here enumerated can be cured until the curvatures of the spine have been corrected.

How can this cure be effected?

Unfortunately, the majority of those seeking the true answer, are still hopelessly groping in the dark after having read more or less false and true literature and listened to more or less false or true advice pertaining to this subject, or by reason of the fact that they could neither afford the time necessary nor the expense incidental to such methods advocated which might have proved beneficial to them. Comparatively few of these seekers have learned the truth and benefited from it.

It is urged that the properly constituted authorities in our research laboratories and health departments impartially investigate the statements herein set forth, to the end that they may solve human ailments by methods of prevention and correction, rather than by methods of "cure." That is what my method of physical education does. I can convince you.

Time and progress are synonymous terms - nothing can stop them - the truth will prevail!

My work will be established and when it is, I will be the happiest man in God's Universe. My goal will have been reached.

Chapter 10: New Style Beds and Chairs

It is scarcely believable in this day and age of revolutionary discoveries and inventions, that the constituted authorities of our Public Health Departments are so deplorably ignorant on the subject of scientifically constructed beds, couches and chairs of all types primarily designed to promote normal health.

That the correctness of the writer's theories in this regard is unqualifiedly supported by other reputable professional and lay investigators, it is only necessary to refer to the mass of pertinent information which he has accumulated during the course of his many years of activity devoted to the keen study and close research of general health problems. The conclusions reached by these various authorities as set forth in this booklet, are fully confirmed by my personal theoretical and practical investigations along these and similar lines.

This prevailing universal lack of understanding of natural laws of health, particularly by professional health authorities is astounding. In fact, it is unique in comparison with the remarkable progressive "Seven League Boot" strides of medical science, mechanization of industry, telephony, radio, television and so on infinitum ad libitum.

The vital statistics of our leading insurance companies indicate unmistakably that the death rate arising from heart disease is constantly increasing. Should not this alarming factor emphasize the urgent necessity for an immediate and intensive study of the underlying causes responsible for this most unfavorable and really unnecessary condition?

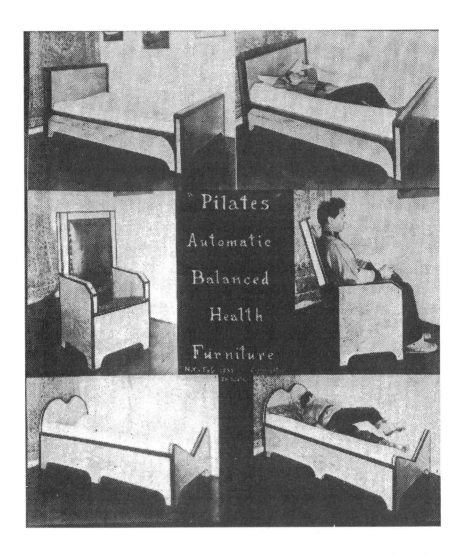

Here are a few more models of my corrective, restful comfort chairs and beds - each made by me in my studio. They can be made up in any kind of wood and any color to fit the color scheme of the most beautiful home.

While it is only too true that heart disease is not infrequently "acquired" in childhood, it is only too true that it is not often discovered until later on in life. Usually, the persons afflicted find it out when between forty to fifty-five years of age; unfortunately, often at a time too late to offer its victims a cure.

Today our public health and research programs do not sufficiently stress the importance due to a profound study of the "laws of mechanics" as applied to the human body. Particularly is this true with reference to a proper consideration and deep study of the necessity for recognition of the importance of the attainment of normal equilibrium of the body in motion, at rest or in sleep.

From a strict humanitarian rather from a purely commercial viewpoint, a close and unbiased study of the reasons responsible for the invariable restless tossing experienced by the average sleeper, can lead to but one definite conclusion with reference to our modern beds - i. e., that while admittedly they are appealing to the eye from an esthetic standpoint and apparently seemingly comfortable, they are, however, as a matter of fact, quite unnatural and impractical for the very purposes that they are supposed to have been originally designed. They do not afford maximum rest and complete relaxation. All they do is to afford a place upon which to toss the body.

Those beds may look pretty, but they absolutely fail in their aid to rest and health.

I have invented a bed that affords both rest and comfort, but the makers of our beautiful beds, will not give my inventions the recognition they deserve, for they fully realize that when this is done, the field of bed manufacturing will be revolutionized.

It is, of course, axiomatic that restful sleep is impossible without the fullest and complete relaxation of all our muscles.

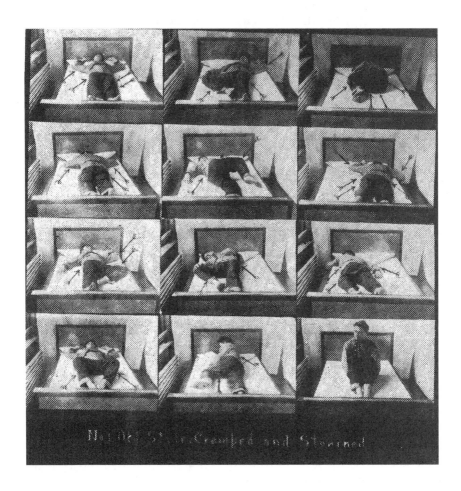

No. Do 5 - Cramped and Strained

Here is the old style bed or the kind almost everyone is using today. The arrow shows the strained position in our present day straight beds. No matter how pretty a bed might be, it cannot and does not give you the comfort and rest of my "V" shape bed. There is nothing but continuous restlessness in the present day bed. All of the chairs and beds illustrated in this book were made by me, from carpentry to upholstery and each model is protected by patents registered with U.S. Patent Office.

Strange as it may seem, to those who are not technically informed, beds equipped with even the very finest of wire bed springs, actually defeat this very object.

Why? Because the bony structure forming the "foundation" of our body does not in beds so equipped receive the necessary natural resistance to afford the requisite simultaneous relaxation of both the skeletal and muscular systems of the human body.

Under these adverse circumstances, the body has, so to speak, literally to snatch rest with its corresponding motion of relaxation "on the fly," as it were. I have taken motion pictures of a person in sleep covering a period of eight hours, and my film, the same of that of the outstanding manufacturer of beds today, records as many as forty-five different changes of position during sleep. In fact, mine showed 48, and his, 45. In my bed, you won't change half a dozen times.

While recognizing the fact that we tire either by too little or by much activity - there is a happy medium - not too much and not too little. Is not an average of $5^5/_8$ movements an hour during sleep rather excessive for persons supposedly enjoying normal health.

Can the body under such conditions really receive the benefit naturally inherent in proper rest which is implied by minimum rather than maximum changes of position during normal sleep?

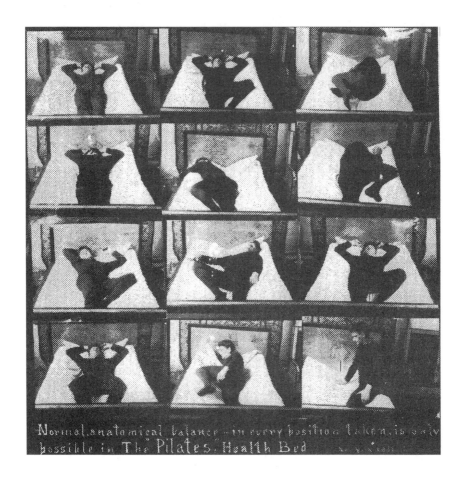

Normal anatomical balance - in every position taken, is only possible in The Pilates Health Bed

Here is the author resting comfortably in one of the bed inventions. Note the manner in which he rests - like the cat or the dog in his natural, comfortable position. This is my "V" shape bed and has been specially devised for the child as a bed for correcting faulty posture and perfect relaxation of the spine and the muscles surrounding it. This "V" bed is especially adopted for the expectant mother, who requires all the comfort and rest she can get and also requires a perfect spine. This is the natural bed for the hospital for expectant mothers, asthma sufferers and consumptives.

Is it not perfectly reasonable and logical to deduce from this inference that our present-day beds are unfortunately neither designed nor constructed to afford the maximum of proper rest for the body? This deduction is demonstrably true. Here are the facts:

From time immemorial, it has been the stupid parents, wholly ignorant of the laws of nature, who have unknowingly inflicted needless cruelty upon their offspring. They have labored under the false impression that their growing children must stretch their little legs out straight while sleeping in their beds instead of permitting them to retain the natural and normal position in sleep. That normal position is one in which they entered the world. It is a position similar to that taken by the cat family and other animals when they curl themselves up in a "coil," just before going to sleep.

In this respect, it would seem that the instinct of the mothers of the animal kingdom is to that extent, at least, far superior to the unthinking practice of the mothers of mankind. Unfortunately, this is only one instance of the many "sins" against the laws of nature committed by the majority of mothers calculated to jeopardize the present health and future welfare of their progeny. Certainly if animals thrive on such coiling practice, mankind can do likewise. Try it and see for yourself. You won't suffer from constipation, weak kidneys and other ailments if you sleep as the cat sleeps.

Why haven't our educators the moral courage to advocate the immediate destruction of all the old and musty orthodox tomes which continue to perpetuate the teaching of false health doctrines? Why don't they actively advocate the immediate substitution therefore of modern physical culture books based upon sane, sound and safe methods such as I have preached in this book? Do you want the answer? It is because such adoption would ruin them.

Why does practically every one naturally assume, what might be for want of a better term, called the "kitten coil" position when preparing to go to sleep?

Why do health authorities assert that to assume this natural position is not only unnatural but also not conducive to good health?

What sound, logical arguments can be advanced to support the obvious falsity of the latter foregoing conclusion?

Is it correctly based upon any well known and equally well recognized principles governing the laws of nature?

Why is it that children and adults alike, whenever opportunity presents itself, invariably tend when seated to lean backward in a tilted position and balance themselves on the rear legs of a chair?

Why do mothers and fathers object to the foregoing practice (aside from the fact that doing so, scratches the chair and mars the wall etc.)?

Why do most of us become more or less restless and lean backward and forward, cross our legs from left to right and vice versa after we have been sitting in a chair for only a comparatively short period of time?

Why is it that it is more comfortable to "squat" on the floor, Turkish or American Indian fashion, than it is to sit comfortably for a longer or shorter time in an ordinary chair?

Why are present-day chairs and beds not what they should be - mediums for rest, relaxation and normal sleep?

The correct answers to the foregoing series of closely related questions are all of paramount importance and should be closely studied. You have them all in this book.

I will be most happy to demonstrate my system and my inventions to all interested. My aim is to offer a real service to humanity from an altruistic and philanthropic point of view.

I am not of the mercenary, quack type. I welcome the opportunity to furnish further detailed information regarding my personal views on the subject of "Tension" and "Relaxation" as related to the attainment and maintenance of normal health to all who read this.

I have the only course in the world that teaches physical education on a corrective basis and brings the results I claim for it. I have invented, as I already stated, several variety of chairs - one for the kindergarten children to build proper posture and keep the spine as God intended it to be; another for the benefit of those afflicted with knock-knees, bow-legs and flat feet, also a corrective chair; still another for the development of proper posture for the man who must sit at a desk and has little time for exercising; and a fourth as an aid for those who have been afflicted with the scourge of infantile paralysis and require leg and arm movements.

I have invented, as I have already stated, several types of beds and mattresses, which, those who have viewed them in my studios at 939 Eighth Avenue, have marveled at. Those beds and mattresses are so revolutionary, that when I showed a model to a leading bed and mattress manufacturer with the aim of having him produce them in quantities, his chief engineer remarked:

"Prof. Pilates, your invention is marvelous, but it cannot be adopted by us because if we did, it would mean turning our entire plant topsy-turvy. We would have to destroy all of our present-day models and create new advertising and that would practically mean starting out on a new business."

And immediately following that, this firm began to advertise extensively the very thing I had submitted - namely, that a person in sleep moves from forty to fifty times, and that by the use of their specially constructed mattress, such restlessness is reduced at least thirty percent. But do they? Certainly not! They still sell and use the old style mattress and bed. It was just a ruse to offset any advertising I might do.

What folly! I appeal in this book to those interested in the future welfare of our race.

I appeal to them to aid in putting my practical physical education method before the public where it will do most benefit, and to have them see and test my health producing inventions to the end that mankind can enjoy God's blessing - health and happiness.

Part II

1945 Edition of

Joseph Pilates'

Return to Life through Contrology

Introducing Part II and Fitness Principles Evolved from Contrology

Eleven years after Joseph Pilates first published his thoughts on exercise, in _Your Health_, he published _Return to Life through Contrology_, his continuing theories of exercise. This time, however, he also included his fundamental 34 exercises with photographic sequences and step by step instructions. Many students and instructors have read his words carefully and reiterated the fundamentals of fitness as heard in his opening words and in his careful design of his starter set of exercises.

Pilates himself further evolved and developed his own exercises over the following years. He also developed intricate equipment for use in addition to or in place of his basic matwork exercises seen in _Return to Life through Contrology_. It was only natural that, with the growing popularity of Pilates' exercises, owing to both publicity and effectiveness, the 21st Century would see fitness specialists who would continue Pilates' own thinking and progress. Others would realize that using additional equipment, both simple and complex, could augment and enhance the fundamentals learned in Pilates' only two books.

Return to Life through Contrology begins with the opening sentence: "Physical fitness is the first requisite of happiness." His long, opening chapter of this book is quite obviously a continuation of his thoughts and writings from _Your Health_. He presents and then supports the thesis that "the basic fundamentals of a natural physical Education" must begin with the realization that civilization impairs physical fitness but that his program of Contrology can restore it. His guiding principles have now been elucidated by many writers. His own words offer memorable images of water flowing through mountain streams. He draws metaphorical parallels to our own blood circulation that provides the same cleansing effects within our own bodies.

Each section of the opening chapter in this second book of his clarifies for the reader a bit more of Pilates' thinking. He explicitly paints a world view that achieving the highest accomplishments within the scope of our capabilities in all walks of life depends on constantly striving to acquire strong, healthy bodies at the same time as developing our minds to the limit of our ability. He leads an interested reader directly toward the group of 34 exercises found in _Return to Life through Contrology_. In the same way, this set of starter exercises has led generations of fitness enthusiasts into new exercises, using new tools and new approaches, in the 21st Century.

It has become common practice to teach Pilates' theories as being founded on six fundamental principles of exercise: Breathing, Centering, Concentration, Control, Flow, and Precision. In Return to Life through Contrology, Pilates writes that:

> **Breathing** is the first act of life, and the last. Our very life depends on it. Since we cannot live without breathing it is tragically deplorable to contemplate the millions and millions who have never learned to master the art of correct breathing.

This is so patently obvious. Our own instructional cues emphasize it greatly. Our reading of his words would place breathing first among the six, even if it weren't already first in alphabetical order.

Even in Pilates' original exercise instructions, you will find extraordinary instructional emphasis on inhalations and exhalations. Pilates continually emphasized that students should use very full, deep breaths. He used the metaphor of a bellows being much like our lungs; we should expand and contract our lungs in a full, complete and similar way to pump the air fully in and out of the body.

The other five fundamentals that are drawn from his words merely underlie all subsequent fitness fundamentals and exercise designs. It is more valuable to understand how these six principles integrate with one another and, in total, account for the great effectiveness of Pilates' exercises and the resultant combination of strength, grace, balance, and ease that one experiences as a result.

Centering represents the act of drawing your own mental and physical focus during each exercise to the core, or center (often called the 'powerhouse', of your body. This is roughly the area between your lower ribs and hips, although it also includes the lower and upper back muscles.

Concentration is simply paying close attention to the specifics and details of every Pilates exercise. Bring your full attention to the movements of each exercise in order to obtain maximum value. Pilates' words are:

> "Concentrate on the correct movements EACH TIME YOU EXERCISE, lest you do them improperly and thus lose all the vital benefits of their value. Correctly executed and mastered to the

point of subconscious reaction, these exercises will reflect grace and balance in your routine activities. Contrology exercises build a sturdy body and sound mind fitted to perform every daily task with ease and perfection as well as to provide tremendous reserve energy for sports, recreation, emergencies.

You can see here how Pilates returns over and over again to the body and mind connection, and to the benefits of his program in all the things we experience in daily life: His words resonate repeatedly with the Greek concepts of body *and* mind:

Control represents the concept that it is your mind that directs and manages each separate muscular movement.

Be certain that you have your entire body under complete mental control... Good posture can be successfully acquired only when the entire mechanism of the body is under perfect control.

Flow is a just a lovely word that has been extracted from Pilates' writings about Pilates exercise that can and should be done in a flowing manner, with the goals of fluidity, elegance, and grace. The intention is that the energy one exerts during each exercise should connect all body parts smoothly and thereby flow evenly through your body.

Precision is the final fundamental principle and for the technically inclined among us, it is imperative that we as students maintain, and we as instructors teach, a conscious awareness of precision during each exercise's movements. Pilates' original teachings and step by step instructions were always very specific in the placement, alignment, and trajectory for each moving part of the body.

It's a wonderful foundation from a century ago for all the recent and ongoing evolution of Pilates' principles into so many interesting, effective and novel new fitness programs and techniques. Continue reading now to see precisely what Joe touted nearly 100 years ago. Part III in this book will later demonstrate where evolution has brought us in the 21st Century.

Pilates Return to Life through Contrology

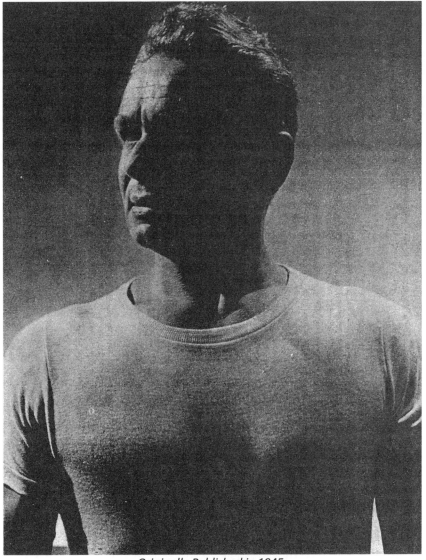

Originally Published in 1945:
by Joseph H. Pilates *and* William John Miller

Pilates' Return to Life Through Contrology

Originally Published in 1945 as:

Return to Life
Through Contrology

by Joseph H. Pilates *and* William John Miller

Edited, Reformatted and Reprinted
in a New Easy-to-Read Edition
by Presentation Dynamics
949-666-5030
http://www.JosephPilates.org

Photographs of Joseph H. Pilates at sixty

Updated with a New Introduction by
Judd Robbins and Lin Van Heuit-Robbins

ACKNOWLEDGMENT

The authors appreciate this opportunity to express thanks to all loyal friends and students for their sustained encouragement which cheered them onward in the preparation of this book. Special gratitude is acknowledged to Beatrice E. Rogers for most valuable assistance rendered, and to George Hoyningen-Huene for his unusual patience and exceptional professional skill in the production of the fine photography illustrating the technical text throughout RETURN TO LIFE.

DEDICATION

to "Clara"

INTRODUCTION by Joseph Pilates

MORTAL perfection is achievable only through bodily perfections and therefore the development of physique to high levels of strength and beauty, under control of the mind. This is the first requisite of human achievement Also the maintenance of a superior standard of physical fitness is increasingly necessary to the maintenance of life and liberty in any complex civilization. It is supremely so in times of social strife. Therefore, the discovery and use of the most efficient programs of physical improvement are now vital to the very preservation of the race.

In my judgment, Contrology is an ideal system to transform the body into a perfect instrument of the will. It is kinesiologically proper, physiologically sound, and psychologically correct. I have personal knowledge of its success in effecting astonishing results, not only for normal adults but also for those suffering from supposedly incurable physical defects and organic deficiencies.

For twenty years, I have studied professionally the leading systems of body development proposed and used in schools, colleges, private gymnasia, and other institutions, and have no hesitation in saying that the Pilates system is not merely 20 or 50 or 80 per cent more efficient, but must be several times as effective as any practicable combination of other systems.

To appreciate the truth of this statement the reader must himself have experimented with other systems, and then must have actually used Contrology. For it develops not only the muscles of the body, suppleness of the limbs, and functioning of vital organs and endocrine glands; it also clarifies the mind and develops the will.

So it is with great pleasure that I endorse Joseph H. Pilates' work, and hope it will spread throughout our country, bringing increased physical fitness to all.

Frederick Rand Rogers
President
North American Physical Fitness Institute

INTRODUCTION by Judd Robbins and Lin Van-Heuit Robbins

Certified Trainers in The Matwork
Developed by Joseph and Clara Pilates
And Owner-Managers of
http://JosephPilates.org
A centralized resource on the Internet for students and trainers alike interested in the latest worldwide developments relating to the influential work of Joseph H. Pilates. At this site, you can and learn from the growing band of students and trainers who are spreading the word and building on the foundation of exercises developed originally by Joseph and Clara Pilates.

This new printing of Joseph Pilates' original 1945 work retains the original photographs and step-by-step poses and accompanying instructions. While some of the latest research in the fitness world might suggest caution when performing some of these poses and exercises, the overall program of exercises developed at the turn of the 20th Century remains astoundingly effective and beneficial for fitness enthusiasts in the 21st Century.

As with all exercise programs, you should consult your doctor before commencing to follow any or all of the exercises and poses presented in this book. The overall impact of Joseph Pilates' exercises can be extraordinarily beneficial to anyone suffering from a variety of physical weaknesses. However, the exercises are most effective when presented to beginners by a trainer who has studied the matwork instructions as well as the fundamental physiological and biomechanical aspects of the body so analytically coordinated into the exercises by Joseph Pilates.

Table Of Contents – Original Return to Life through Contrology

Basic Fundamentals of a Natural Physical Education **95**

Civilization Impairs Physical Fitness...95

Contrology Restores Physical Fitness..98

Guiding Principles of Contrology 100

Bodily House-cleaning with Blood Circulation 101

Results of Contrology..110

The Original Exercises **113**

1. The Hundred... 114

2. The Roll Up... 116

3. The Roll-Over With Legs Spread (Both Ways) 118

4. The One Leg Circle (Both Ways) 120

5. Rolling Back 122

6. The One Leg Stretch 124

7. The Double Leg Stretch... 126

8. The Spine Stretch.. 128

9. Rocker With Open Legs... 130

10. The Cork-Screw 132

11. The Saw 134

12. The Swan-Dive.. 136

13. The One Leg Kick 138

14. The Double Leg Kick.. 140

15. The Neck Pull.. 142

16. The Scissors... 144

17. The Bicycle 146

18. The Shoulder Bridge 148

19. The Spine Twist 150

20. The Jack Knife... 152

21. The Side Kick 154

22. The Teaser.. 156

23. The Hip Twist With Stretched Arms............................. 158

24. Swimming 160

25. The Leg-Pull — Front 162

26. The Leg-Pull... 164

27. The Side Kick Kneeling 166

28. The Side Bend... 168

29. The Boomerang... 170

30. The Seal 172

31. The Crab.. 174

32. The Rocking.. 176

33. The Control Balance 178

34. The Push Up 180

The Basic Fundamentals of a Natural Physical Education
(from Joe's original Return to Life Through Contrology)

CIVILIZATION IMPAIRS PHYSICAL FITNESS

Physical fitness is the first requisite of happiness. Our interpretation of physical fitness is the attainment and maintenance of a uniformly developed body with a sound mind fully capable of naturally, easily, and satisfactorily performing our many and varied daily tasks with spontaneous zest and pleasure. To achieve the highest accomplishments within the scope of our capabilities in all walks of life we must constantly strive to acquire strong, healthy bodies and develop our minds to the limit of our ability. This very rapidly progressing world with its ever-increasing faster tempo of living demands that we be physically fit and alert in order that we may succeed in the unceasing race with keen competition which rewards the "go-getter" but by-passes the "no-getter."

Physical fitness can neither be acquired by wishful thinking nor by outright purchase. However, it can be gained through performing the daily exercises conceived for this purpose by the founder of Contrology whose unique methods accomplish this desirable result by successfully counteracting the harmful inherent conditions associated with modern civilization.

In the Stone Age and onward man lived mostly outdoors with practically little shelter from the elements. He has not yet lived long enough indoors with protection against the elements to be able to successfully withstand the daily strains and stresses imposed upon him by our present mode of "fast" living. This explains why both you and I and all the rest of us are compelled in our own interest to give constant thought to the improvement of our bodies and to spend more time in acquiring and maintaining that all-important goal of physical fitness.

All in all, we do not give our bodies the care that our well-being deserves. True, we do stroll in the fresh air whenever our whimsical spirit moves us, or whenever necessity compels us to do so, with the result that on these occasions we do, in spite of ourselves, exercise our legs to this limited extent, accomplished, however, at the sacrifice of the rest of our body which after all is much more important to us from the viewpoint of our general health. Is it any wonder then that this haphazard and wholly inadequate body-building technique of the average person fails so miserably in the acquirement of physical fitness!

Admittedly, it is rather difficult to gain ideal physical fitness under the handicap of daily breathing the soot-saturated air of our crowded and noisy cities. On the other hand, we can more quickly realize this ambition if we are privileged to breathe the pure fresh air of the country and forests without the accompaniment of the traffic roar of the city which constantly tends to keep our nerves strung taut. Even those of us who work in the city and are fortunate enough to live in the country must counteract the unnatural physical fatigue and mental strain experienced in our daily activities. Telephones, automobiles, and economic pressure all combine to create physical letdown and mental stress so great that today practically no home is entirely free from sufferers of some form of nervous tension.

Because of the intense concentration demanded by our work and despite the real enjoyment our work may bring some of us we, nevertheless, gladly welcome any additional relief in the form of diversified and pleasant recreational activities, preferably outdoors, in our constant attempts to offset the effects of increasing cares and burdens so common today. To ease mental strain and relieve physical fatigue we must acquire a reserve stockpile of nervous energy in order that we may really be able to enjoy ourselves at night.

Hobbies and all forms of play tend materially to renew our vitality with accompanying moral uplift. Play is not necessarily only confined to indulging in conventional games. Rather the term "play" as we use it here, embraces every possible form of pleasurable living. For example, simply spending a quiet and pleasant evening at home with our family chatting with congenial friends is, according to our interpretation, a form of play that is delightful, pleasant social entertainment as distinguished from our daily work. This finds us cheerful, contented, and relaxed.

However, many of us at the end of our daily work lack sufficient energy at night for recreation. How many of us simply spend the night routinely reading the evening newspaper? How many of us are entirely too exhausted to read, even occasionally, an interesting book, visit our friends, or see one of the latest motion pictures?

When some of us occasionally spend a weekend away from our usual city haunts and environments, instead of receiving the immediate benefits of that desirable change in the way of complete revitalization (without fatigue) as the result of our experience outdoors in the bright sunshine, we are more often than not likely to find ourselves only recovering from the shock of our disappointment about the middle of the following week.

Why? Because our previous mode of living and the consequent neglect of our bodies has not prepared us for reaping the beneficial results of this diversion. We lacked the necessary reserve energy to draw upon for this purpose and the fault lies only with us and not with nature as most of us like to think. All that any normal body should require is a change from whatever it has previously been subjected to.

Accordingly, since we are living in this Modern Age we must of necessity devote more time and more thought to the important matter of acquiring physical fitness. This does not necessarily imply that we must devote ourselves only to the mere development of any particular pet set of muscles, but rather more rationally to the uniform development of our bodies as a whole - keeping all our organs as nearly as possible in their naturally normal condition so that we may not only be in a better position to earn our daily bread but also so that we may have sufficient vitality in reserve at night for the enjoyment of compensating pleasure and relaxation.

Perhaps with some feeling of doubt you ask, "How can I realize such a utopian condition? At night I am much too tired to go to a gymnasium." Or, "Isn't it too costly to enroll for a conditioning course in some good gymnasium or club?" RETURN TO LIFE fully explains how you can successfully achieve your worthy ambition to attain physical fitness right in your own home and at only nominal cost.

CONTROLOGY RESTORES PHYSICAL FITNESS

Contrology is complete coordination of body, mind, and spirit. Through Contrology you first purposefully acquire complete control of your own body and then through proper repetition of its exercises you gradually and progressively acquire that natural rhythm and coordination associated with all your subconscious activities. This true rhythm and control is observed both in domestic pets and wild animals - without known exceptions.

Contrology develops the body uniformly, corrects wrong postures, restores physical vitality, invigorates the mind, and elevates the spirit. In childhood, with rare exceptions, we all enjoy the benefits of natural and normal physical development. However, as we mature, we find ourselves living in bodies not always complimentary to our ego. Our bodies are slumped, our shoulders are stooped, our eyes are hollow, our muscles are flabby and our vitality extremely lowered, if not vanished. This is but the natural result of not having uniformly developed all the muscles of our spine, trunk, arms, and legs in the course of pursuing our daily labors and office activities.

If you will faithfully perform your Contrology exercises regularly only four times a week for just three months as outlined in RETURN TO LIFE, you will find your body development approaching the ideal, accompanied by renewed mental vigor and spiritual enhancement. Contrology is designed to give you suppleness, natural grace, and skill that will be unmistakably reflected in the way you walk, in the way you play, and in the way you work. You will develop muscular power with corresponding endurance, ability to perform arduous duties, to play strenuous games, to walk, run or travel for long distances without undue body fatigue or mental strain. And this by no means is the end.

One of the major results of Contrology is gaining the mastery of your mind over the complete control of your body. How many beginners are amazed and chagrined (even trained athletes in the public eye) to discover how few (if any) Contrology exercises they are able to execute properly! Their previous failure to exercise regularly and properly, or their method of training, has not helped them.

There is unmistakable evidence, too, that the functioning of the brain has correspondingly deteriorated. The brain itself is actually a sort of natural telephone switchboard exchange incorporated in our bodies as a means of communication through the sympathetic nervous system to all our muscles.

Unfortunately, pure reason plays only a minor part in the lives of most of us. In practically every instance the daily acts we perform are governed by what we THINK we see, hear, or touch, without stopping first to analyze or think of the possible results of our actions, good or bad. As the result of habit or reflex action, we wink, dodge, and operate machines more or less automatically. IDEALLY, OUR MUSCLES SHOULD OBEY OUR WILL. REASONABLY, OUR WILL SHOULD NOT BE DOMINATED BY THE REFLEX ACTIONS OF OUR MUSCLES. When brain cells are developed, the mind too is developed. Teachers start with sense organs. Contrology begins with mind control over muscles.

By reawakening thousands and thousands of otherwise ordinarily dormant muscle cells, Contrology correspondingly reawakens thousands and thousands of dormant brain cells, thus activating new areas and stimulating further the functioning of the mind. No wonder then that so many persons express such great surprise following their initial experience with Contrology exercises caused by their realization of the resulting sensation of "uplift." For the first time in many years their minds have been truly awakened. Continued use of Contrology steadily increases the normal and natural supply of pure rich blood to flow to and circulate throughout the brain with corresponding stimulation to new brain areas previously dormant. More significantly, it actually develops more brain cells. G. Stanley Hall, the great American psychologist, observed:

"The culture of muscles is brain-building."

Contrology is not a fatiguing system of dull, boring, abhorred exercises repeated daily "ad-nauseam." Neither does it demand your joining a gymnasium nor the purchasing of expensive apparatus. You may derive all the benefits of Contrology in your own home. The only unchanging rules you must conscientiously obey are that you must always faithfully and without deviation follow the instructions accompanying the exercises and always keep your mind wholly concentrated on the purpose of the exercises as you perform them. This is vitally important in order for you to gain the results sought, otherwise, there would be no valid reason for your interest in Contrology. Moreover, you must accept all collateral advice with equal fidelity. Remember that you are teaching yourself - right! The benefits of Contrology depend solely upon your performing the exercises exactly according to instructions - and not otherwise.

Remember, too, that "Rome was not built in a day," and that PATIENCE and PERSISTENCE are vital qualities in the ultimate successful accomplishment of any worthwhile endeavor. Practice your exercises diligently with the fixed and unalterable determination that you will permit nothing else to sway you from keeping faith with yourself. At times you may feel tempted to "take a night off." Don't succumb to this momentary weakness of indecision, or rather, wrong decision. Decide to remain true to yourself. Think of what would happen if the stokers firing the boilers of a giant ocean liner were to decide to "take a night off."

You know the answer. If they were to repeat this action, you know the result. The human body, fortunately, can withstand more neglect, successfully, than can the complicated machinery of a modern steamship. However, that is no good reason why we should unnecessarily and unreasonably tax our bodies beyond bounds of endurance, especially since doing so results only in hurting ourselves. Schopenhauer, the philosopher, said: "To neglect one's body for any other advantage in life is the greatest of follies."

Make up your mind that you will perform your Contrology exercise ten minutes without fail. Amazingly enough, once you travel on this Contrology "Road to Health" you will subconsciously lengthen your trips on it from ten to twenty or more minutes before you even realize it. Why? The answer is simple: The exercises have stirred your sluggish circulation into action and to performing its duty more effectively in the matter of discharging through the bloodstream the accumulation of fatigue - products created by muscular and mental activities. Your brain clears and your will power functions.

BODILY HOUSE-CLEANING WITH BLOOD CIRCULATION

This is the equivalent of an "internal shower." As the spring freshets born of the heavy rains and vast masses of melting snows on mountains in the hinterlands cause rivers to swell and rush turbulently onward to the sea, so too will your blood flow with renewed vigor as the direct result of your faithfully performing the Contrology exercises. These exercises induce the heart to pump strong and steadily with the result that the bloodstream is forced to carry and discharge more and more of the accumulated debris created by fatigue.

Contrology exercises drive the pure fresh blood to every muscle fibre of our bodies, particularly to the very important capillaries which ordinarily are rarely ever fully stimulated once we have reached adulthood. As a heavy rainstorm freshens the water of a sluggish or stagnant stream and whips it into immediate action, so Contrology exercises purify the blood in the bloodstream and whip it into instant action with the result that the organs of the body, including the important sweat glands, receive the benefit of clean fresh blood carried to them by the rejuvenated bloodstream. Observe the beneficial effects that Contrology exercises have on your heart action.

Contrology exercises guard against unnecessary pounding or throbbing of your heart. Study carefully the poses illustrated by the photographs and note that all the exercises are performed while you are in a sitting or reclining position. This is done to relieve your heart from undue strain as well as to take advantage of the more normal (original) position of the visceral organs of your body when in such positions. Contrary to exercises performed in an upright position, those performed while you are in a recumbent position do not aggravate any possible undetected organic weakness.

True heart control follows correct breathing which simultaneously reduces heart strain, purifies the blood, and develops the lungs. To breathe correctly you must completely exhale and inhale, always trying very hard to "squeeze" every atom of impure air from your lungs in much the same manner that you would wring every drop of water from a wet cloth. When you stand erect again, the lungs will automatically completely refill themselves with fresh air.

This in turn supplies the bloodstream with vitally necessary life-giving oxygen. Also, the complete exhalation and inhalation of air stimulates all muscles into greater activity. Soon the entire body is abundantly charged with fresh oxygen, a fact which makes itself instantly known as the revitalized blood reaches the tips of your fingers and toes similarly as the heat generated by a good head of steam in your boiler and properly distributed by your radiators is felt in every room in your house.

Breathing is the first act of life, and the last. Our very life depends on it. Since we cannot live without breathing it is tragically deplorable to contemplate the millions and millions who have never learned to master the art of correct breathing. One often wonders how so many millions continue to live as long as they do under this tremendous handicap to longevity. Lazy breathing converts the lungs, figuratively speaking, into a cemetery for the deposition of diseased, dying, and dead germs as well as supplying an ideal haven for the multiplication of other harmful germs.

Therefore, above all, learn how to breathe correctly. "SQUEEZE" EVERY ATOM OF AIR FROM YOUR LUNGS UNTIL THEY ARE ALMOST AS FREE OF AIR AS IS A VACUUM. Stand erect again and observe how your lungs will automatically completely refill themselves with fresh air. The impact of so much oxygen upon your bloodstream may at first quite naturally and normally result in your experiencing a slight sensation of "lightheadedness," similar to the effect you might experience were you for the first time to find yourself actively engaged in the rarefied atmosphere high up in the mountains. However, after a few days this feeling will entirely disappear.

Whenever you read the word "rolling" in the exercises, be sure to hold your chin pressed tightly against your chest and, when you lie down or when you rise, "roll" and "unroll," your spine exactly in imitation of a wheel rolling forward and backward. Vertebra by vertebra try to "roll" and "unroll" as suggested. It is this very action of "rolling" and "unrolling" that cleanses your lungs so effectively by driving out the impure air and forcing in the pure air as you "roll" and "unroll." Indefatigably and conscientiously practice breathing until the art of correct breathing becomes habitual, automatic and subconscious, which accomplishment will result in the bloodstream receiving its full quota of oxygen and thus ward off undue fatigue.

Study carefully. Do not sacrifice knowledge to speed in building your solid exercise regime on the foundation of Contrology. Follow instructions exactly as indicated down to the very smallest detail. There is a reason! Contrology is not a system of haphazard exercises designed to produce only bulging muscles. Just to the contrary, it was conceived and tested (for over forty-three years) with the idea of properly and scientifically exercising every muscle in your body in order to improve the circulation of the blood so that the bloodstream can and will carry more and better blood to feed every fibre and tissue of your body.

Nor does Contrology err either by over-developing a few muscles at the expense of all others with resulting loss of grace and suppleness, or at a sacrifice of the heart or lungs. Rather, it was conceived to limber and stretch muscles and ligaments so that your body will be as supple as that of a cat and not muscular like that of the body of a brewery-truck horse, or the muscle-bound body of the professional weight-lifter you so much admire in the circus.

Concentrate on the correct movements EACH TIME YOU EXERCISE, lest you do them improperly and thus lose all the vital benefits of their value. Correctly executed and mastered to the point of subconscious reaction, these exercises will reflect grace and balance in your routine activities. Contrology exercises build a sturdy body and sound mind fitted to perform every daily task with ease and perfection as well as to provide tremendous reserve energy for sports, recreation, emergencies.

Very interesting, but quite obvious when you stop to think of it, is the indisputable fact that no one modern activity employs all our muscles. The nearest approach to this ideal is found in all-round swimming and fancy diving. Walking, the only exercise activity common to most of us, employs only a limited number of muscles. With repetition the art of walking becomes a subconscious habit, not infrequently a bad one, and only too often accompanied by poor posture - note our letter-carriers.

However, there is another important reason for consistently exercising all our muscles; namely, that each muscle may cooperatively and loyally aid in the uniform development of all our muscles. Developing minor muscles naturally helps to strengthen major muscles. As small bricks are employed to build large buildings, so will the development of small muscles help develop large muscles. Therefore, when all your muscles are properly developed you will naturally perform your work with minimum effort and maximum pleasure.

On a pleasant sunshiny morning, how we all naturally thrill in anticipation of accompanying congenial friends on a trip over modern highways to the country in a perfect-running automobile with a good driver at the wheel, knowing that his gradual acceleration and deceleration and his skillful negotiation of even sharp curves and abrupt turns are all accomplished so smoothly that we never give a conscious thought to his fine driving but rather concentrate on enjoying the passing scenery. How different, however, our reactions when taking a similar ride in a neglected car driven by a bad driver whose jerky starts, sudden stops, and dangerous turns not only upset our balance constantly but also rob us of the pleasure of the trip, especially after we realize that, luckily for us, he just missed "capsizing" the car although he did not succeed in avoiding dumping us into the ditch.

With the foregoing examples to guide us, we should wisely select as our pattern of life in this Modern Age that which excludes constant pushing, shoving, rushing, crowding, and wild scrambling all so characteristic of our day. This too fast pace is plainly reflected in our manner of standing, walking, sitting, eating, and even talking and results in our nerves "being on edge" from morning to night and actually depriving us of our needed sleep.

Constantly keep in mind the fact that you are not interested in merely developing bulging muscles but rather flexible ones. Bulging muscles hinder the attainment of flexibility because the over-developed muscles interfere with the proper development of the under-developed muscles. True flexibility can be achieved only when all muscles are uniformly developed. Normal muscles should function naturally in much the same manner as do the muscles of animals.

For instance, at the very next opportunity, watch a cat as it lazily opens its eyes, slowly looks around, and gradually prepares to rise after a nap. First, it gradually rises on its hindquarters and then gradually lowers itself again, at the same time sprawling out on the floor, leisurely stretching its forepaws (with extended claws) and legs. Observe closely how all its back muscles actually ripple as it stretches and relaxes itself. Cats as well as other animals acquire this ideal rhythm of motion because they are constantly stretching and relaxing themselves, sharpening their claws, twisting, squirming, turning, climbing, wrestling, and fighting. Also observe, too, how cats sleep - utterly relaxed whether they happen to be lying on their back, side or belly. Contrology exercises emphasize the need for this constant stretching and relaxing.

Before proceeding, we must speak of the spinal column with which are associated practically all the major activities of our body. The spine is composed of 26 vertebrae. Each vertebra is separated from the other by intervertebral cartilage. This cartilage acts as a cushion to absorb the shock of sudden jars, reduces friction to a minimum, and gives the spine its characteristic flexibility, thus permitting it to function even more freely.

The 'science' of Contrology disproves that prevalent and all-too-trite saying, "You're only as old as you feel." The 'art' of Contrology proves that the only real guide to your true age lies not in years or how you THINK you feel but as you ACTUALLY are as infallibly indicated by the degree of natural and normal flexibility enjoyed by your spine throughout life. If your spine is inflexibly stiff at 30, you are old; if it is completely flexible at 60, you are young.

Because of poor posture, practically 95 per cent of our population suffers from varying degrees of spinal curvature, not to mention more serious ailments. In a newly-born infant the back is flat because the spine is straight.

Of course, we all know that this is exactly as intended by nature not only then but also throughout life. However, this ideal condition rarely obtains in adult life. When the spine curves, the entire body is thrown out of its natural alignment - off balance. Note daily the thousands of persons with round, stooped shoulders, and protruding abdomens. The back would be flat if the spine were kept as straight as a plumb line, and its flexibility would be comparable to that of the finest watch spring steel.

Fortunately, the spine lends itself quite readily to correction. Therefore, in the reclining exercises, be sure wherever indicated, to keep your back full length always pressed firmly against the mat or floor. When rising from the floor or lowering yourself to the floor, always do so with a "rolling" or "unrolling" motion exactly in imitation of a wheel, equipped with imaginary "vertebrae" rolling forward or backward. Vertebra by vertebra try to "roll" and "unroll." These "rolling" and "unrolling" movements tend to gradually but surely restore the spine to its normal at-birth position with its correspondingly increased flexibility. At the same time you are completely emptying and refilling your lungs to their full capacity. This admittedly requires persistence and earnest effort but it is worth it!

It would be a grave error to assume that even Contrology exercises alone will remake a man or a woman into an entirely physically fit person. To understand this statement better, just remember that exercises as such with relation to physical fitness are somewhat similar to the relationship a grindstone or hone bears to an axe or razor. For example, how obvious is the answer to the foolish question as to which of two equally expert woodchoppers would cry "Timber" first, the one with a dull axe or saw, or the one who habitually sharpens his tools nightly in preparation for his work the next day. Correspondingly, proper diet and sufficient sleep must supplement our exercise in our quest for physical fitness. Another important factor in this connection is that of relaxation at stated fixed intervals throughout our workday wherever it is possible to do so, since this practice keeps us physically fit after we have obtained physical fitness. The man who uses intelligence with respect to his diet, his sleeping habits, and who exercises properly, is beyond any question of doubt taking the very best preventive medicines provided so freely and abundantly by nature.

By all means never fail to get all the sunshine and fresh air that you can. Remember too, that your body also "breathes" through the pores of your skin as well as through your mouth, nose, and lungs. Clean, open skin pores permit perspiration to uninterruptedly eliminate the poisons of your body. Moreover, unless you are really chilly, do not exercise in sweatshirts or even in lighter clothing. Whenever and wherever possible, wear "shorts" or sun suits outdoors, and let the life-giving ultraviolet rays reach and penetrate into every skin pore of your body. Do not fear the cold of winter. When you are outdoors wear rather loose-fitting clothes in preference to tight-fitting garments, not overlooking, of course, the importance of stout, comfortable shoes. Breathe properly, walk correctly, and swing along briskly. If you follow this sound advice you will find yourself feeling comfortable and invigorated.

The principal point to remember with regard to diet is to eat only enough food to restore the "fuel" consumed by the body and to keep enough of it on hand at all times to furnish the extra energy required on occasions beyond our normal needs and to meet unexpected emergencies. Merely eating to satisfy one's lust for good food is both foolish and dangerous to one's health. Such a person cannot ever be truly physically fit. No wonder! Youth and growing children quite naturally require a greater intake of food than do adults and the aged. The former are maturing; the latter have matured.

Not only the amount of food but also the kind is largely dependent upon one's occupation and sometimes, lack of it. Is it not reasonable to conclude that the sedentary indoor worker requires proportionately less food and of a different kind than the laborer who is engaged in hard manual toil outdoors? Heavy eating followed immediately by sitting, or even lying down awake or asleep, is comparable to over-loading the firebox with coal and then closing the drafts of the furnace. The former instance is ideal for generating "poisons" that eventually find their way into your bloodstream. The latter instance is ideal if your aim is to maintain a smoldering fire without adequate heat instead of a bright, glowing fire to radiate its comforting warmth throughout your house. You have the choice in either case.

Common sense dictates that you will make the right one. A man eating a heavy meal and indulging in vigorous activity will react thereto comparably to the way that a furnace with drafts open will react to a fire in a well-filled firebox. Accordingly, it is earnestly suggested that you guide your eating habits with all due respect to the required amount of food and kind you need to keep yourself physically fit, always as indicated by your occupation, or lack of it.

Often men, who have been accustomed to work hard on a farm or play hard in school athletics or labor hard in a factory, continue eating the hearty meals they then ate even though now they are engaged only in sedentary indoor occupations where moderate meals are indicated. This practice is very unwise since it unnecessarily adds excess weight to their bodies, much of it in the form of undesirable fat which, if man were a hibernator, he could draw on in much the same manner that hibernating animals do in the winter when they draw against the stockpile of reserved energy with which the instinct of nature has provided them over the long period of their enforced inactivity and "sleep."

Since man is not a hibernating creature, such excess of fat is a real detriment to him, imposing an unnecessarily heavy burden on his heart, liver, bladder and other vitally important organs of his digestive system. Still worse for him is the unnatural formation and accumulation of fat directly around the heart itself. The carrying of this extra poundage produces needless fatigue.

Imagine yourself, for instance, carrying a well-filled traveling bag weighing 20 pounds. For one or two blocks, all goes comparatively well, but with each additional block it is carried, the urge to rest is proportionately increased until at length the resulting fatigue compels you to do so. How relieved you feel after you have reached your final destination! You are doing exactly the very same thing when you persist in carrying 20 needless pounds of excess weight on your body only you are not so keenly aware of it because the weight is carried by the entire body instead of by your carrying arm alone as in the case of the bag. However, fatigue is created thereby in either case. Why not relieve yourself of this truly "excess baggage?"

Once acquired, it is, unfortunately, not so easy to rid yourself of excess weight. Nevertheless, it can be done! Consult your family physician for regular physical check-ups, and then follow his sound advice and instructions implicitly. Every adult over 40 years of age should not deny himself the benefits of a medical examination every three months. Once a year should suffice for younger persons unless some condition indicates to the contrary. Even in their case, consulting their physician twice a year would be wise. If this sound suggestion is followed, latent ailments can be discovered in their early developmental stage, and the "growth" of a long and perhaps serious illness may thus be "nipped in the bud."

If any particular part of your body is under-developed or shows an accumulation of excess fat, select Contrology exercises specifically to correct the respective conditions, repeating the exercises at stated intervals throughout the workday whenever it is possible to do so. However, be sure NEVER TO REPEAT THE SELECTED EXERCISE(S) MORE THAN THE PRESCRIBED NUMBER OF TIMES since more harm will result than good by your unwittingly or intentionally disregarding this most important advice and direction. Why? Because this infraction creates muscular fatigue - poison. There is really no need for tired muscles. Judicious selection of special Contrology exercises will accomplish more for your health and bodily condition, in conjunction with the foregoing advice, than all else combined.

Now let us consider the important question of good sleep at night. A quiet, cool, well-ventilated room is best. Do not use a soft mattress. "Firm but not soft" is a good rule to follow. Use the lightest possible bed covering consistent with warmth. Do not use large bulky pillows (or as some do, two stacked pillows) - better still, use none at all.

Most important in the matter of enjoying good recuperative sleep are quiet, darkness, fresh air, and mental calm. Nervousness is usually aggravated by a lack of proper exercise, especially in the case of one with a troubled mind. The best alleviative for this condition is exercise. So if your sleep is disturbed, rise immediately and perform your exercises. It is far better to be tired from physical exertion than to be fatigued by the "poisons" generated by nervousness while lying awake. Particularly beneficial in this regard are the spinal "rolling" and "unrolling" massage exercises which relax the nerves and induce sound, restful sleep.

While conceding the fact that nowadays practically every one of us routinely indulges in daily baths, experience has nevertheless taught us that only a small minority really achieve thorough cleanliness thereby, from our point of view. In our opinion, the correct technique to use in accomplishing this highly desirable result is to use only a good stiff brush (no handle) since this type of brush forces us to twist, squirm, and contort ourselves in every conceivable way in our attempts to reach every portion of our body which is otherwise comparatively easy to reach with a handle brush.

The use of a good stiff brush as described stimulates circulation, thoroughly cleans out the pores of the skin and removes dead skin too. The pores of your skin must "breathe" - they cannot do so unless they are kept open and freed from clogging. Your skin will soon respond most gratifyingly to this perhaps seemingly "Spartan-like" treatment and acquire in the process a new, fresh, glowing appearance, and develop a texture smooth and soft to the touch. So brush away merrily, and heartily too!

Finally, beginning with the introductory lesson, each succeeding exercise should be mastered before proceeding progressively with the following exercises. Make a close study of each exercise and do not attempt any other exercise until you first have mastered the current one and know its routine down to the last detail without any reference to the text. Be certain that you have your entire body under complete mental control.

RESULTS OF CONTROLOGY

Good posture can be successfully acquired only when the entire mechanism of the body is under perfect control. Graceful carriage follows as a matter of course. Just as a good smooth-running automobile engine is the result of proper parts correctly assembled so that it operates with a minimum consumption of gasoline and oil with comparatively little wear, so too is the proper functioning of your own body the direct result of the assembled Contrology exercises that produce a harmonious structure we term physical fitness reflecting itself in a coordinated and balanced tri-part unity of body, mind, and spirit. This in turn results in perfect posture when sitting, standing, or walking with the utilization of approximately only 25 per cent of your energy while the approximately remaining 75 per cent in the form of surplus energy reserve is "on call" to meet the needs of any possible emergency.

The art of correct walking consists principally and simply in a slight tilting forward of the proper standing posture, alternately placing one foot before the other with the weight of the body poised and balanced on the balls of the feet. Be careful not to lock your knees as doing so will jar the spine and interrupt the rhythmic walking motion.

Standing also is very important and should be practiced at all times until it is mastered. First, assume the correct posture, then when tired, shift the weight of the body from one side to the other while resting on the "idle" side. Do not push your hips out or lock your knees. Progress forward with a slightly swaying graceful motion comparable to the effect created by a gentle breeze blowing over a field of growing wheat ready for harvest, causing it to gracefully sway in "waves" from its roots to its tips. Never slouch, as doing so compresses the lungs, overcrowds other vital organs, rounds the back, and throws you off the balance created by poising the weight of your body on the balls of your feet.

If you will faithfully follow the instructions, beginning with the introductory lesson, you will without doubt acquire correct physical fitness with proper mental control. You will truly be building upon the solid foundation of Contrology which itself is built upon scientific principles so true, sound and unique that the science and art of Contrology will live forever.

As you progress in your self-instruction, you never have anything to "unlearn." These exercises will actually become a part of your very self securely stored away forever in your subconscious mind. You who have learned correctly how to ride a bicycle, how to swim, or how to drive an automobile need never worry with respect to the possibility of your failing to use the right technique in these skills on all occasions because of the confidence born of the fact that you realize you received your instructions from the best available source and authority. So, too, the acquirement and practice of the art and science of Contrology will instill that confidence in you that will remain forever for future use as occasions therefore may indicate. Then it is simply only a question of "re-toning" the muscles that have in the meantime become "soft" as the result of disuse.

With body, mind, and spirit functioning perfectly as a coordinated whole, what else could reasonably be expected other than an active, alert, disciplined person? Moreover, such a body freed from nervous tension and over-fatigue is the ideal shelter provided by nature for housing a well-balanced mind that is always fully capable of successfully meeting all the complex problems of modern living. Personal problems are clearly thought out and calmly met.

The acquirement and enjoyment of physical well-being, mental calm and spiritual peace are priceless to their possessors if there be any such so fortunate living among us today. However, it is the ideal to strive for, and in our opinion, it is only through Contrology that this unique trinity of a balanced body, mind, and spirit can ever be attained. Self-confidence follows.

The ancient Athenians wisely adopted as their own the Roman motto: "Mens sana in corpore sano" (A sane mind in a sound body). And the Greeks as a people displayed even greater wisdom when they practiced what they preached and thus came nearest to achieving its actual accomplishment. Self-confidence, poise, consciousness of possessing the power to accomplish our desires, with renewed lively interest in life, are the natural results of the practice of Contrology. Thus we achieve happiness, for is not real happiness truly born of the realization of worthwhile work well done, with the gratification of enjoying the other pleasures flowing from successful accomplishment with its compensating measure of "play" and resulting relaxation?

So in your very commendable pursuit of all that is implied in the trinity of godlike attributes that only Contrology can offer you, we bid you not good-bye but "au revoir" firmly linked with the sincere wish that your efforts will result in well-merited success chained to everlasting happiness for you and yours.

THE EXERCISES

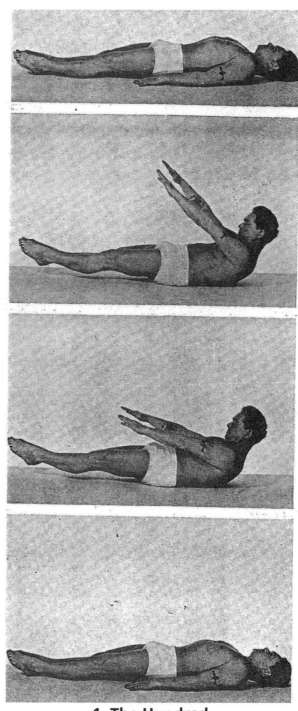

1. The Hundred

INSTRUCTIONS for "The Hundred"

Pose 1   (a) Take position illustrated
                (b) Lie flat with body resting on mat or floor
                (c) Stretch arms (shoulder-wide, touching body, palms down) straight forward
                (d) Stretch legs (close together, knees locked) straight forward
                (e) Stretch toes (pointed) forward and downward

Pose 2   (a) INHALE SLOWLY
                (b) Lift both feet about 2" above mat or floor
                (c) Raise head with eyes focused on toes
                (d) Raise both arms about 6" to 8" above thighs

Pose 3   (a) EXHALE SLOWLY
                (b) Raise and lower both arms (tensed)
                (c) From shoulders only
                (d) Without touching body
                (e) Within a radius of 6" to 8"
                (f) Mentally counting 5 movements while
                (g) EXHALING SLOWLY
                (h) Alternating with 5 similar movements while
                (i) INHALING SLOWLY
                (j) Begin with only 20 movements and
                (k) Gradually increase them in units of
                (1) 5 additional movements each time until a
                (m) Maximum of 100 movements is reached
                (n) Never exceed 100 movements

Pose 4   (a) Relax completely

REMARKS

At first you probably will not be able to carry out instructions as illustrated in poses - this proves why these exercises and all succeeding ones will benefit you. However, with patience and perseverance you eventually should succeed in achieving the ideals as posed - with accompanying normal health.

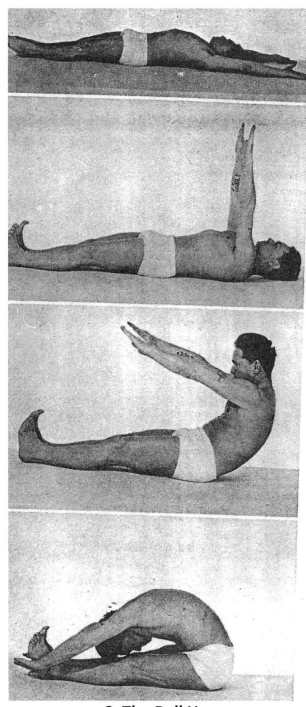

2. The Roll Up

INSTRUCTIONS for "The Roll Up"

Pose 1   (a) Lie flat with entire body resting on mat or floor
(b) Stretch arms (shoulder-wide, palms up) straight backward
(c) Stretch legs (close together. knees locked) straight forward
(d) Stretch toes (pointed) forward and downward

Pose 2   (a) Begin INHALING SLOWLY and bring arms (shoulder-wide) straight forward to upright right angle position and
(b) Toes (pointed) upward

Pose 3   (a) While still INHALING SLOWLY
(b) Bend head forward and downward until
(c) Chin touches chest and then
(d) Begin EXHALING SLOWLY and
(e) Start "rolling" slowly upward and straight forward

Pose 4   (a) While EXHALING SLOWLY finish
(b) "Rolling" forward until
(c) Forehead touches legs and then
(d) Begin INHALING SLOWLY while returning to Pose 3 and Poses 2 and 1

NOTE:

Repeat the foregoing exercise three (3) times, trying with each repetition not only to stretch the entire body more and more but also to reach farther and farther straight forward as indicated.

CAUTIONS

Pose 1 - Entire spine must touch mat or floor. Tense body (do not bend arms or legs).

Pose 3 - Press both legs against mat or floor; if at first unsuccessful, placing cushion on your feet will materially help you.

Pose 4 - Legs must remain flat on mat or floor (knees locked). Palms must remain flat on mat or floor (arms stretched straight forward).

REMARKS

This exercise strengthens the abdominal muscles and restores the spine to normal.

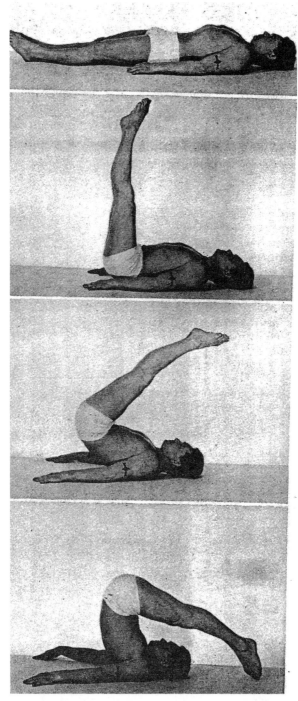

3. The Roll-Over with Legs Spread (Both Ways)

INSTRUCTIONS for "The Roll-Over"

Pose 1   (a) Take position illustrated

           (b) Lie flat on mat or floor

           (c) Stretch arms (shoulder-wide, touching body, palms down) straight forward

           (d) Stretch (close together, knees locked) straight forward

           (e) Stretch toes (pointed) forward and downward

Poses   (a) INHALE SLOWLY and

2-3-4   (b) Begin raising legs upward and over until

           (c) Toes touch mat or floor

           (d) EXHALE SLOWLY and

           (e) Press arms firmly against mat or floor

           (f) Spread legs as far apart as possible

Poses   (a) INHALE SLOWLY and

4-3-2   (b) Begin "rolling" slowly downward with

           (c) Both legs (tensed) straight (and spread as for apart as possible)

           (d) Until spine touches mat or floor

           (e) EXHALE SLOWLY while

Pose 1   (a) Returning to position 1

           (b) With legs about 2" above mat or floor

NOTE

Repeat foregoing exercise five (5) times with legs close together at the start of first movement and five (5) times with legs spread apart as far as possible at the start of the second movement.

CAUTIONS

Pose 3 - Keep legs (tensed, knees locked) as far apart as possible. Roll downward slowly from one vertebra to another.

Pose 4 - Keep back and head firmly pressed to mat or floor.

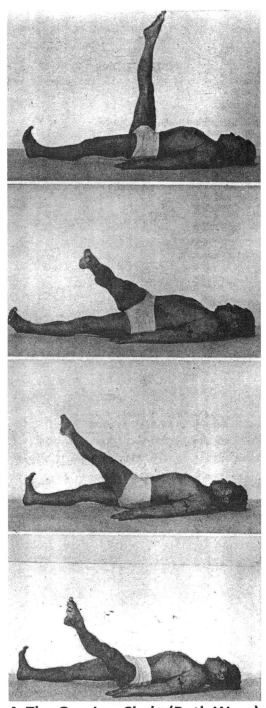

4. The One Leg Circle (Both Ways)

INSTRUCTIONS for "The One Leg Circle"

Pose 1   (a) Lie flat with entire body resting on mat or floor
               (b) Stretch arms (shoulder-wide, touching body, palms down) straight forward
               (c) Bring right leg to upright right angle position
               (d) Stretch toes (pointed) forward and downward
               (e) Left toes upward

Pose 2   (a) Begin EXHALING SLOWLY at start of downward motion with right leg while making a complete left-to-right circle (in the air) over the left thigh, then
               (b) Begin inhaling slowly at start of upward motion with right leg in completing this circle
               (c) Begin exhaling slowly at start of downward motion with left leg while making a complete right-to-left circle (in the air) over the right thigh, then
               (d) Begin inhaling slowly at start of upward motion with left leg in completing this circle

Pose 3 and Pose 4   (a) Begin inhaling slowly at start of upward motion and with left leg while making a complete right-to-left circle (in the air) over the right ankle, then
               (b) Begin exhaling slowly at start of downward motion with left leg in completing this circle
               (c) Begin inhaling slowly at start of upward motion with right leg while making a complete left-to-right circle (in the air) over the left ankle, then
               (d) Begin exhaling slowly at start of downward motion with right leg in completing this circle

NOTE

Repeat the foregoing exercise five (5) times with each leg.

CAUTIONS

Pose 1 - Toes must be pointed forward and downward (knee locked), right leg. Keep left leg (knee locked) flat on mat or floor with toes "pulled" upward and backward. Shoulders and head must always remain flat on mat or floor.

Pose 2 - Same as Pose 1 but note that right hip is raised.

Pose 4 - Same as Pose 2 but note that left hip is raised. "Swing" left and right legs as far as possible when making circles. Shoulders and head must always remain flat on mat or floor.

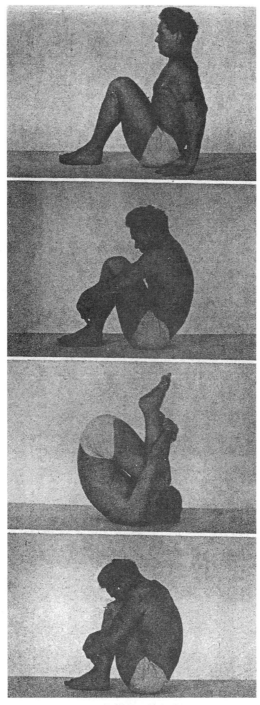

5. Rolling Back

INSTRUCTIONS for "Rolling Back"

Pose 1   (a) Take position illustrated
Pose 2   (a) Grasp legs tightly with locked arms
              (b) Try to press thighs to chest
              (c) Bend head forward and downward with chin touching chest
              (d) Toes (pointed) forward and downward
              (e) INHALE SLOWLY
              (f) "Rock" backward to Pose 3 position
Pose 3   (a) EXHALE SLOWLY while
              (b) Returning to Pose 2 position

NOTE

Repeat the foregoing exercise six (6) times.

CAUTIONS

Pose 2 - Press chest in, round back, head down; keep feet off mat or floor.

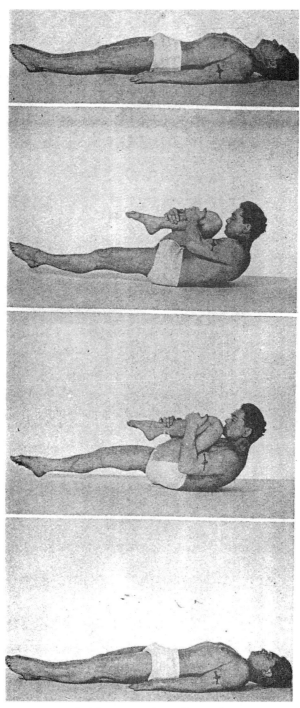

6. The One Leg Stretch

INSTRUCTIONS for "The One Leg Stretch"

Pose 1 (a) Lie flat with entire body resting on mat or floor
Pose 2 (a) Bend head forward until
            (b) Chin touches chest, then
            (c) While INHALING SLOWLY clasp hands and
            (d) "Pull" right leg as far as possible toward chest
            (e) Keep left leg stretched forward (knee locked)
            (f) Stretch toes (pointed) forward and downward with
            (g) Heel raised (about 2")
Pose 3 (a) While EXHALING SLOWLY
            (b) Clasp hands and
            (c) "Pull" left leg as far as possible toward chest
            (d) Keep right leg stretched forward (knee locked)
            (e) Stretch toes (pointed) forward and downward with
            (f) Heel raised (about 2")

NOTE

Repeat the foregoing exercise five (5) times with each leg. (Later on the number of repetitions may be gradually and progressively safely increased to twelve (12) times with each leg.)

CAUTIONS

Pose 2 - Chin must touch chest. You must see your toes. Heels must be raised (about 2").

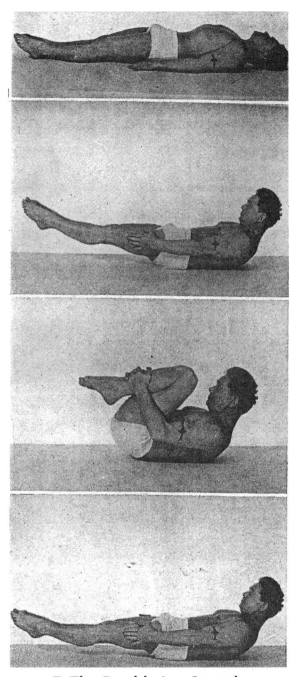

7. The Double Leg Stretch

INSTRUCTIONS for "The Double Leg Stretch"

Pose 1	(a) Take position illustrated
	(b) Rest entire body on mat or floor
	(c) Legs (close together) straight forward
	(d) Knees locked
	(e) Toes (pointed) forward and downward
	(f) Arms stretched straight forward beside body
	(g) Palms down
Pose 2	(a) INHALE SLOWLY
	(b) Head up
	(c) Chin to chest
	(d) Arms stretched straight forward and
	(e) Pressed firmly against thighs
	(f) Heels raised about 2" off mat or floor
	(g) Palms inward
Pose 3	(a) EXHALE SLOWLY
	(b) "Draw" both legs upward and forward and with
	(c) Locked wrists hold them firmly in "doubled-up" position as indicated
	(d) "Pull" legs toward you and press them firmly against chest
Pose 4	(a) INHALE SLOWLY

NOTE

Repeat the foregoing exercise six (6) times. Later to twelve (12).

CAUTIONS

Pose 2 - Head pressed firmly against chest. Abdomen in. Heels raised about 2" off mat or floor.

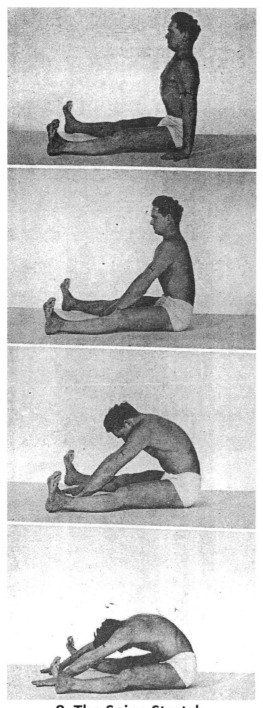

8. The Spine Stretch

INSTRUCTIONS for *"The Spine Stretch"*

Pose 1   (a) Take position illustrated
                (b) Spread legs as wide apart as possible
                (c) "Draw" toes (pointed) upward and backward

Pose 2   (a) Rest palms flat on mat or floor, then with
                (b) Outstretched arms, palms flat on mat or floor
                (c) Chin touching chest
                (d) Begin reaching forward with three (3) successive "sliding" motion-stretching movements as far forward as possible until you assume position as illustrated in Poses 3 and 4

NOTE

Repeat the foregoing exercise three (3) times, trying with each repetition to reach farther and farther forward as indicated.

CAUTIONS

Pose 4 - Continue EXHALING SLOWLY, abdomen "drawn" in, chin pressed firmly against chest.

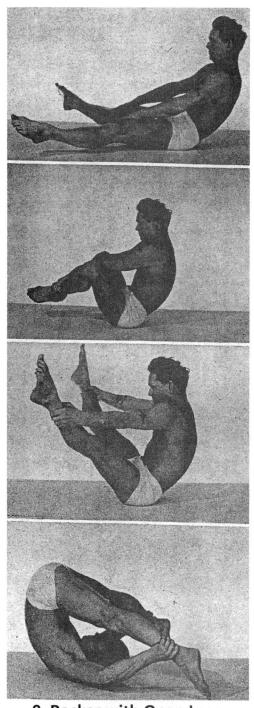

9. Rocker with Open Legs

INSTRUCTIONS for "Rocker with Open Legs"

Pose 1   (a) Take position illustrated
Pose 2   (a) Bend knees
            (b) INHALE SLOWLY
Pose 3   (a) Grasp ankles firmly
            (b) Toes (pointed) forward and downward (knees locked)
            (c) Spread legs upward and outward as far as possible
            (d) Keep abdomen "drawn" in as far as possible with
            (e) Chin touching chest
Pose 4   (a) EXHALE SLOWLY
            (b) "Roll" over backward trying to touch mat or floor with toes

NOTE

Repeat the foregoing "rocking" exercise backward and forward six (6) times.

CAUTIONS

Pose 3 - Arms and legs rigid (elbows and knees locked). "Pivot" on base of spine, "rocking" backward to Pose A position, then "rock" forward, pressing head firmly against chest, at the same time pressing arms firmly forward against legs until you reach Pose 3 and try to balance yourself in that position.

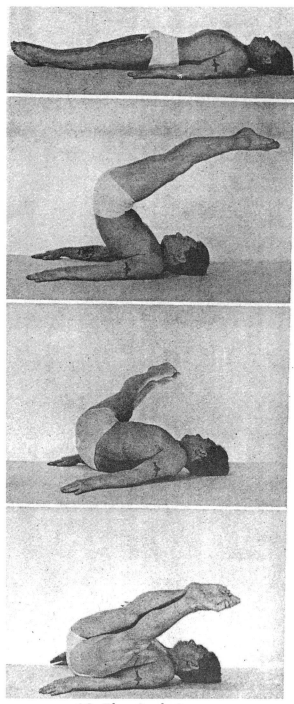

10. The Cork-Screw

INSTRUCTIONS for "The Cork-Screw"

Pose 1   (a) Take position illustrated
                (b) Entire spine must rest on floor or mat
                (c) Arms straight forward touching body
                (d) Palms down

Pose 2   (a) INHALE SLOWLY
                (b) Raise legs (close together) "rolling" upward until
                (c) Body rests on shoulders, arms and head
                (d) Knees locked
                (e) Toes (pointed) forward and downward

Pose 3   (a) EXHALE SLOWLY
                (b) Lower both legs together, but not to mat or floor
                (c) Knees locked
                (d) Toes (pointed) forward and downward
                (e) Twist trunk "corkscrew" fashion until
                (f) Body is partially lowered on right side to mat or floor

Pose 4   (a) INHALE SLOWLY
                (b) Make a complete right-to-left circle upward as far
                      as possible and return to Pose 2 position

Pose 3   (a) EXHALE SLOWLY
                (b) Lower both legs together but not to mat or floor
                (c) Knees locked
                (d) Toes (pointed) forward and downward
                (e) Twist trunk "corkscrew" fashion until
                (f) Body is partially lowered on left side to mat or floor

Pose 4   (a) INHALE SLOWLY
                (b) Make a complete left-to-right circle upward as far
                      as possible and return to Pose 2 position

NOTE

Repeat the foregoing exercise three (3) times each.

CAUTIONS

Pose 3 and Pose 4 - While "circling" keep both shoulders pressed to mat or floor. Arms straight.

REMARKS

This exercise strengthens neck and shoulders and is an internal and spinal massage.

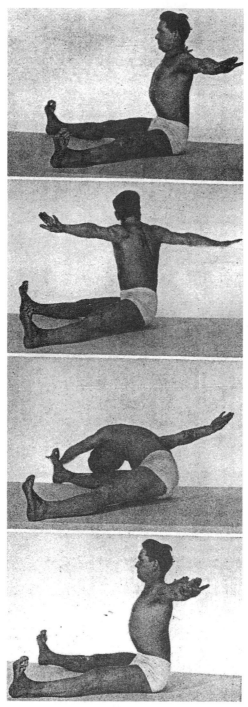

11. The Saw

INSTRUCTIONS for "The Saw"

Pose 1   (a) Take position as illustrated
                    (b) Spread legs as wide apart as possible
                    (c) Head up
                    (d) Chin "drawn" in
                    (e) Chest out
                    (f) Abdomen "drawn" in
                    (g) Arms (shoulder-high) pressed backward until shoulder blades lock
                    (h) INHALE SLOWLY

Pose 2   (a) Twist body (from trunk only) to right as far as possible

Pose 3   (a) Bend forward and downward as far as possible until
                    (b) Left hand crosses and rests diagonally and centrally on right foot
                    (c) EXHALE SLOWLY while
                    (d) Stretching body forward in three (3) successive sliding-reaching "saw-like" motions as far as possible

Pose 4   (a) Resume position illustrated in this pose
                    (b) INHALE SLOWLY

Pose 2   (a) Twist body (from trunk only) to left as far as possible

Pose 3   (a) Bend forward and downward as far as possible until right hand crosses and rests diagonally and centrally on left foot
                    (b) EXHALE SLOWLY while
                    (c) Stretching body forward in three (3) successive sliding-reaching "saw-like" motions as far as possible.

NOTE

Repeat the foregoing exercise three (3) times each.

CAUTIONS

Pose 2 - Twist body before bending forward as in Pose 3.
Pose 3 - Lift raised arm backward and upward as high as possible as indicated in this pose.

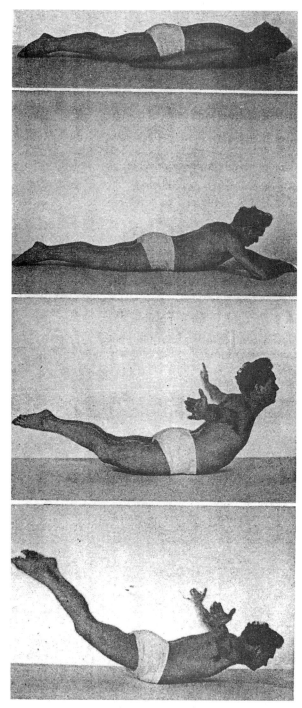

12. The Swan-Dive

INSTRUCTIONS for "The Swan-Dive"

Pose 1   Take position illustrated
and
Pose 2

Pose 3   (a) INHALE SLOWLY
(b) Head raised upward and backward as far as possible
(c) Chest raised high from mat or floor
(d) Raise arms upward and sideward in line with locked   shoulders
(e) Turn palms upward (right to left)
(f) Legs (close together) stretched and raised off mat or floor
(g) Toes (pointed) forward and downward (knees locked)
(h) Body rigid
(i) Back locked

Pose 4   (a) EXHALE SLOWLY as you "rock" forward
(b) INHALE SLOWLY as you "rock" upward

NOTE

Repeat the foregoing "rocking" exercise six (6) times.

CAUTIONS

Pose 3 - Keep back locked, legs off mat or floor, head back, arms rigid, shoulders locked.

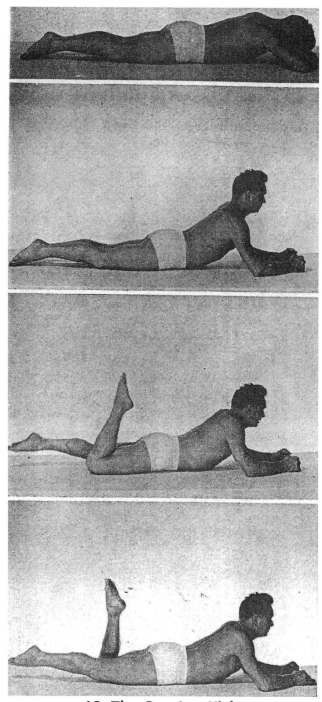

13. The One Leg Kick

INSTRUCTIONS for "The One Leg Kick"

Pose 1   (a) Take position illustrated

                (b) Arms stretched backward

                (c) Firmly pressed to sides of body

                (d) Fists clenched

                (e) Face down and

                (f) Chin touching mat or floor

                (g) Toes (pointed) forward and downward

                (h) Knees locked

Pose 2   (a) Lie on abdomen

                (b) Head up

                (c) Raise chest above mat or floor

                (d) Stretch arms forward to right angle position

                (e) Rest clenched fists on mat or floor

                (f) Stretch legs (close together) straight backward

                (g) Keep knees locked

                (h) Toes (pointed) forward and downward

Pose 3   (a) INHALE SLOWLY and

                (b) Raise legs about 2" above mat or floor

                (c) Try to snap-kick heel of right leg to buttocks

Pose 4   (a) EXHALE SLOWLY while

                (b) Stretching right leg backward and with

                (c) Heel of left leg

                (d) Try to snap-kick heel of left leg to buttocks

NOTE

Repeat the foregoing exercise six (6) times - right and left.

CAUTIONS

Pose 2 - Head up. Chest above mat or floor.

Pose 3 - Keep toes (pointed) above mat or floor.

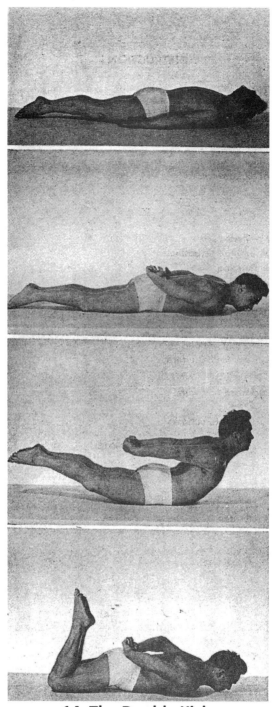

14. The Double Kick

INSTRUCTIONS for "The Double Kick"

Pose 1   (a) Take position illustrated
            (b) Lie flat with head resting on arms
            (c) Stretch legs (close together) straight backward
            (d) Knees locked
            (e) Toes (pointed) forward and downward

Pose 2   (a) Rest chin on mat or floor
            (b) Fold arms backward
            (c) Grasp fingers of left hand with right hand
            (d) Stretch legs (close together) straight backward
            (e) Knees locked
            (f) Toes (pointed) backward and downward and
            (g) Raised about 1" above mat or floor

Pose 3   (a) Raise legs forward to right angle position

Pose 4   (a) INHALE SLOWLY
            (b) Thrust chest out with head thrown back as far as possible and at the same time
            (c) Raise arms (locked) from body
            (d) Stretch backward (tensed) as far as possible, then
            (e) Snap-kick legs (tensed) straight backward and
            (f) Raised as high as possible from mat or floor

NOTE

Repeat foregoing exercise five (5) times.

CAUTIONS

Pose 4 - Keep head up as high as possible. Keep arms stretched backward as far as possible without touching body.

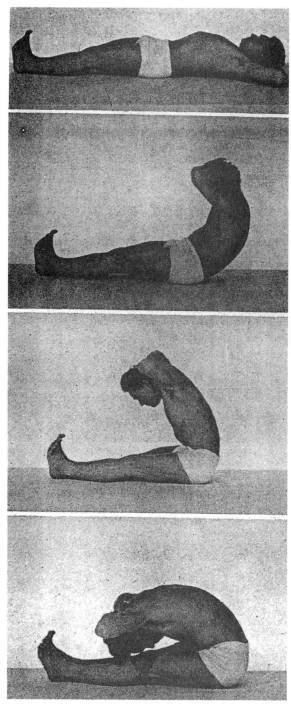

15. The Neck Pull

INSTRUCTIONS for "The Neck Pull"

Pose 1   (a) Take position illustrated
               (b) INHALE SLOWLY
               (c) Clasp hands (fingers firmly interlocked) behind head
               (d) Toes (pointed) up and backward

Pose 2   (a) Bend head forward, chin touching chest
               (b) Abdomen "drawn" in
               (c) Toes (pointed) upward
               (d) Spine "bowed" forward off mat or floor

Pose 3   (a) EXHALE SLOWLY
               (b) Tense and press legs firmly downward against mat or floor
               (c) Slowly raise body upward and forward to position as indicated
               (d) Toes (pointed) upward

Pose 4   (a) EXHALE SLOWLY
               (b) Bend body forward until head and knees meet if possible, as illustrated
               (c) Keep elbows straight backward until shoulder blades lock
               (d) INHALE SLOWLY while
               (e) Returning to Pose 3 position
               (f) EXHALE SLOWLY while
               (g) Returning to Poses 2 and 1 positions

NOTE

Repeat the foregoing exercise three (3) times.

CAUTIONS

Pose 1 - Keep toes (pointed) upward.
Pose 2 - Keep legs pressed firmly to mat or floor (if necessary, placing cushion on feet).
Pose 4 - Elbows straight backward until shoulder blades lock.

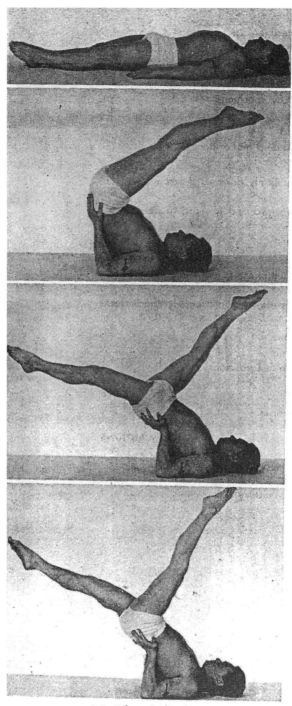

16. The Scissors

INSTRUCTIONS for "The Scissors"

Pose 1   (a) Take position illustrated

Pose 2   (a) Bring legs upward until

              (b) Your body rests on head, shoulders, upper arms, neck and elbows, then with

              (c) "Cupped" hands supporting hips

              (d) INHALE SLOWLY

Pose 3   (a) "Split" legs scissors-like (left leg backward; right leg forward)

              (b) Legs stretched (knees locked)

              (c) Toes (pointed) forward and downward

Pose 4   (a) EXHALE SLOWLY

              (b) Alternate "split" legs scissors-like (right leg backward; left leg forward)

NOTE

Repeat the foregoing scissors - like exercise six (6) times.

CAUTIONS

Pose 2 - Keep body rigid, move legs only, knees locked, toes (pointed) forward and downward. Try gradually to execute "split" so that toes of forward leg, in alternating movements, are beyond your vision; and backward leg, in alternating movements, likewise.

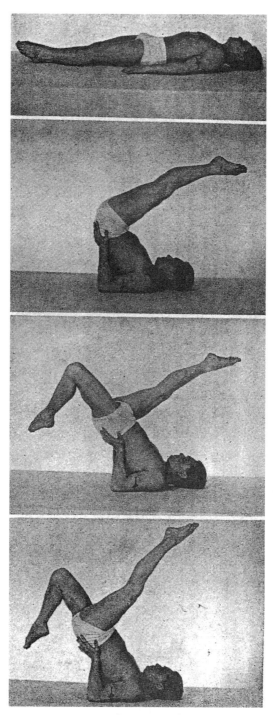

17. The Bicycle

INSTRUCTIONS for "The Bicycle"

Pose 1   (a) Take position illustrated
Pose 2   (a) Raise body on arms, elbows, shoulders, neck, and
             head
             (b) INHALE SLOWLY
             (c) "split" legs (Pose 3)
Pose 3   (a) Bend right knee downward and backward and try
             to "kick" yourself
             (b) EXHALE SLOWLY
Pose 4   (a) "Pull" right leg straight backward
             (b) INHALE SLOWLY
             (c) Bend left knee downward and backward and try to
             "kick" yourself

NOTE
Repeat the foregoing "kicking" exercise five (5) times with each leg.

CAUTIONS
Pose 3 - Be sure to assume position as nearly as possible to that illustrated in this pose. Stretch each leg alternately forward beyond your vision with knee locked, toes (pointed) forward and downward.

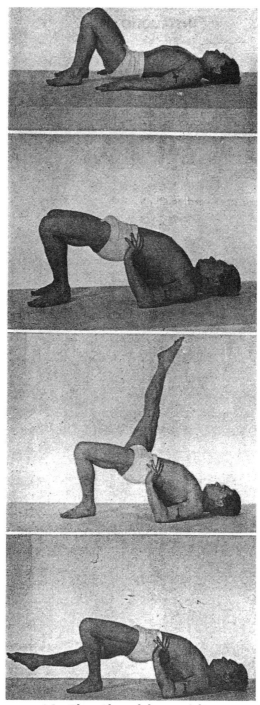

18. The Shoulder Bridge

INSTRUCTIONS for "The Shoulder Bridge"

Pose 1   (a) Take position illustrated

Pose 2   (a) Raise body on upper arms, elbows, shoulders, neck, head, with both feet flat on mat or floor

           (b) Grasp waist firmly with both hands as illustrated

Pose 3   (a) INHALE SLOWLY

           (b) Raise right leg forward and upward to upright position

           (c) Toes (pointed) forward and downward

Pose 4   (a) EXHALE SLOWLY

           (b) Lower right leg forward and downward without bending knee and with knee locked

           (c) Thrust chest upward and outward as far as possible as illustrated in this pose

Pose 3   (a) INHALE SLOWLY

           (b) Raise left leg forward and upward to upright position

           (c) Toes (pointed) forward and downward

Pose 4   (a) EXHALE SLOWLY

           (b) Lower left leg forward and downward without bending knee and with knee locked

           (c) Thrust chest upward and outward as far as possible as illustrated in this pose

NOTE

Repeat left leg and right leg movements three (3) times.

CAUTIONS

Pose 3 - Toes pointed. Knee of right leg is locked. Press foot firmly downward on mat or floor as each leg is lowered and chest thrust out.

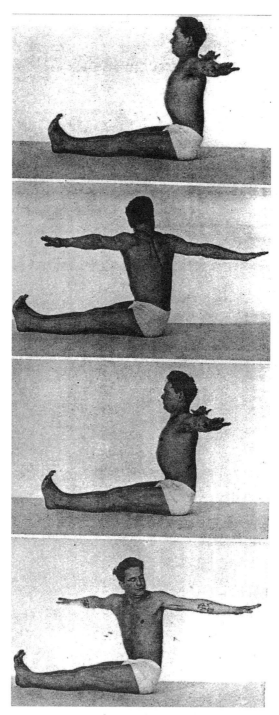

19. The Spine Twist

INSTRUCTIONS for "The Spine Twist"

Pose 1   (a) Take position illustrated
              (b) INHALE SLOWLY
              (c) Sit perfectly upright in right angle position
              (d) Chest out
              (e) Abdomen "drawn" in
              (f) Head up
              (g) Arms (shoulder-wide, palms down) stretched backward until shoulder blades lock
              (h) Legs together, resting full length on mat or floor
              (i) Toes (pointed) upward and backward

Pose 2   (a) Keeping arms and legs absolutely rigid
              (b) EXHALE SLOWLY while
              (c) Twisting body and turning head to right as far as possible, then with two (2) further supreme mental and physical efforts, strive to better your original first attempt
              (d) INHALE SLOWLY while
              (e) Returning to position in

Pose 3   (a) Illustration

Pose 4   (a) EXHALE SLOWLY while
              (b) Twisting body and turning head to left as far as possible, then with two (2) further supreme mental and physical efforts, strive to better your original first attempt
              (c) INHALE SLOWLY while
              (d) Returning to position in

Pose 3   (a) Illustration

NOTE

Repeat the foregoing exercise three (3) times left and three (3) times right, trying with each repetition to reach farther and farther backward.

CAUTIONS

Pose 1 - Keep arms and legs absolutely rigid. Shoulder blades locked. Twist body from spine only. Try to touch chin alternately to right and left shoulder.

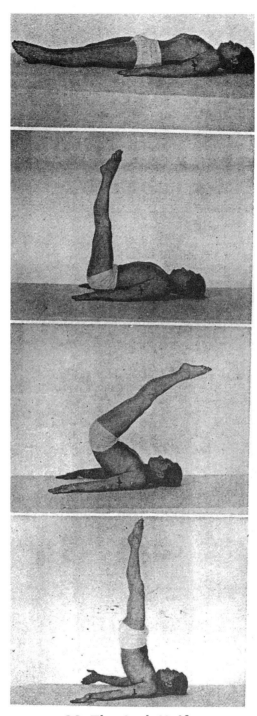

20. The Jack Knife

INSTRUCTIONS for "The Jack Knife"

Pose 1   (a) Take position illustrated
           (b) Rest entire spine on mat or floor

Pose 2   (a) Stretch arms sidewise
           (b) Both legs (close together) raised upward to right   angle position
           (c) Knees locked
           (d) Toes (pointed) forward and downward
           (e) INHALE SLOWLY

Pose 3   (a) Press arms firmly downward against mat or floor
           (b) With knees locked "roll" body over until
           (c) Spine is raised off mat or floor (about 5")

Pose 4   (a) "Kick" legs in snappy "jack-knife" fashion straight upward until
           (b) Entire body rests on head, neck, shoulders, arms
           (c) EXHALE SLOWLY
           (d) Return to Pose 3 position
           (e) INHALE SLOWLY and then
           (f) Return to Pose 2 position
           (g) EXHALE SLOWLY

NOTE

Repeat the foregoing exercise three (3) times.

CAUTIONS

Pose 2 - Keep legs in right angle position, knees locked, toes pointed.
Pose 3 - Hold Pose 3 position for mental count of 2.
Pose 4 - Hold Pose 4 position for mental count of 2.

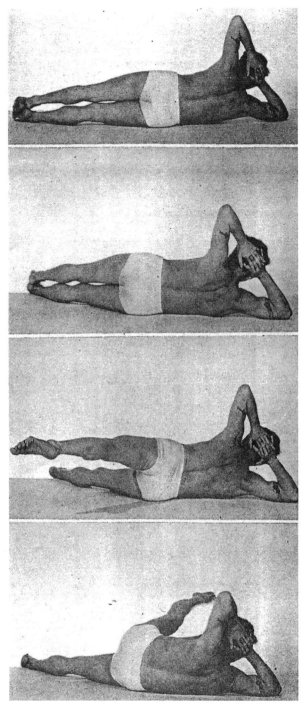

21. The Side Kick

INSTRUCTIONS for "The Side Kick"

Pose 1   (a) Take position illustrated
               (b) Lock hands behind head
               (c) Head up
               (d) Eyes straight forward
               (e) Arms straight in line with shoulders
               (f) Lie full length right side on mat or floor

Pose 2   (a) Bring legs (close together) forward about 2 feet

Pose 3   (a) INHALE SLOWLY
               (b) "Swing" left leg forward as far as possible to you
               (c) Return left leg about 1 foot backward and
               (d) "Swing" left leg forward to you again and attempt
               to better your first trial

Pose 4   (a) EXHALE SLOWLY
               (b) "Swing" left leg backward as far as possible
               (c) Return left leg about 1 foot forward and
               (d) "Swing" left leg backward again and attempt to
                    better your first trial

NOTE

Repeat the foregoing exercise three (3) times, left side. Reverse position of Pose 1, now lying full length on left side on mat or floor. Repeat three (3) additional times, now using your right leg, the sequence of poses 2, 3, and 4.

CAUTIONS

Pose 3 - Head up elbows back. Keep entire body rigid. Move "free" leg only. Keep other leg in straight line pressed against mat or floor.
Pose 4 - Maintain balance lying on side of body.

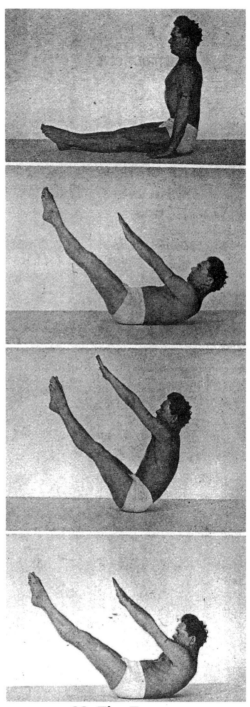

22. The Teaser

INSTRUCTIONS for "The Teaser"

Pose 1   (a) Take position illustrated
              (b) Head up
              (c) Legs (close together)
              (d) Knees locked
              (e) Toes (pointed) forward and downward
              (f) Arms at right angle position beside body
              (g) Hands pointed straight forward
Pose 2   (a) Bend head forward
              (b) Chin to chest
              (c) Press abdomen in
              (d) "Roll" backward on spine until
              (e) Legs are raised upward to indicated angle
Pose 3   (a) INHALE SLOWLY
              (b) Raise arms in parallel line with legs as indicated
Pose 4   (a) "Roll" forward and upward
              (b) "Pivot" on rump keeping
              (c) Raised arms in line with raised legs as indicated
                   (parallel)
              (d) EXHALE SLOWLY and
              (e) Return to Pose 2 position and,
              (f) INHALE SLOWLY

NOTE

Repeat the foregoing exercise three (3) times.

CAUTIONS

Pose 3 - Arms and legs must be kept in straight parallel lines. Keep back well rounded. Chest pressed in.

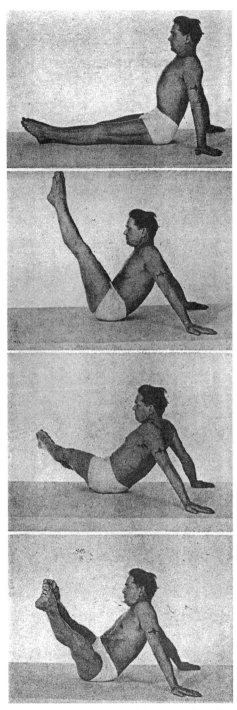

23. The Hip Twist with Stretched Arms

INSTRUCTIONS for "The Hip Twist with Stretched Arms"

Pose 1   (a) Take position illustrated
             (b) Put arms in right angle position
             (c) Firmly pressed to mat or floor with
             (d) Palms of hands in backward position
             (e) Keep legs (close together) straight forward
             (f) Keep toes (pointed) forward and downward

Pose 2   (a) INHALE SLOWLY
             (b) Swing legs (close together)
             (c) Knees lock
             (d) Toes (pointed) forward and downward
             (e) As high as possible

Pose 3   (a) EXHALE SLOWLY on downward
             (b) "Swing" without legs touching mat or floor

Pose 4   (a) INHALE SLOWLY
             (b) "Swing" legs upward as high as possible in right
                  hand circle
             (c) EXHALE SLOWLY and start to
             (d) "Swing" legs downward in left hand circle as far as
                  possible
             (e) Without legs touching mat or floor

NOTE

Repeat the foregoing exercise three (3) times in succession - three (3)
times for left circle, and three (3) times for right hand circle leg "swing"
movements.

CAUTIONS

Pose 1 - Press chest inward as far as possible.
Pose 2 - Chin down.
Pose 4 - When "circling" upward "swing" legs as high and as close to
head as possible. Be sure only legs and hips are moved.

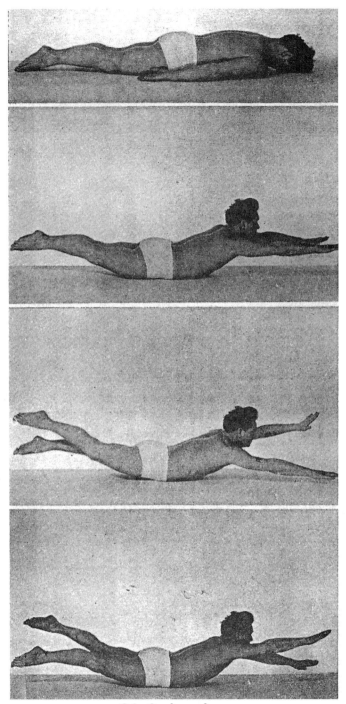

24. Swimming

INSTRUCTIONS for "Swimming"

Pose 1   (a) Take position illustrated
and   (b) Arms stretched forward
Pose 2   (c) Palms down
           (d) Head upward and backward as far as possible
           (e) Chest raised off mat or floor
           (f) Toes (pointed) forward and downward
           (g) Knees locked
           (h) INHALE and EXHALE normally while performing the simultaneous, alternating, compound motions
in   the following movements, counting mentally from
1   to 10, beginning with right arm movement
Pose 3   (a) Left leg and right arm raised upward as far as possible and simultaneously reverse to
Pose 4   (a) Right leg and left arm position and follow instructions under (h) in 2 above

NOTE

Repeat the foregoing exercise as indicated in the preceding instructions.

CAUTIONS

Pose 3 - Left leg and right arm raised as high as possible in upward movements. Left leg and right arm must not touch mat or floor in downward movements. Right leg and left arm raised as high as possible in upward movements. Right leg and left arm must not touch mat or floor in downward movements. Keep body rigid. Move arms and legs only.

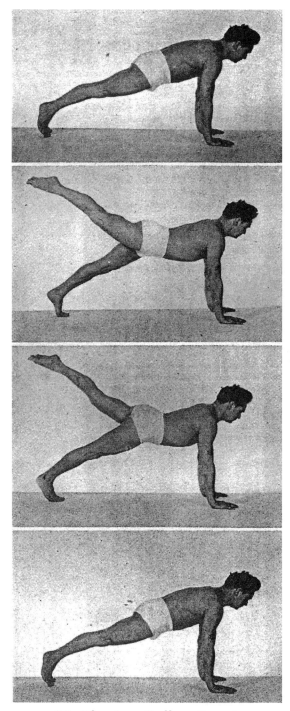

25. The Leg-Pull — Front

INSTRUCTIONS for "The Leg-Pull — Front"

Pose 1   (a) Take position illustrated
                (b) Arms (shoulder-wide) in right angle position
                (c) Hands at right angles
                (d) Head in straight line with body
                (e) Legs close together
                (f) Toes (pointed) downward
                (g) Heels close together
                (h) Knees locked

Pose 2   (a) INHALE SLOWLY
                (b) Raise right leg upward and backward as high as possible
                (c) EXHALE SLOWLY
                (d) Lower right leg to Pose 1 position

Pose 3   (a) INHALE SLOWLY
                (b) Raise left leg upward and backward as high as possible
                (c) EXHALE SLOWLY
                (d) Lower left leg to Pose 1 position

NOTE

Repeat the foregoing exercise three (3) times, right and left.

CAUTIONS

Pose 1 - Arms must be shoulder-wide in right angle position.
Pose 2 - Move legs only, knees locked.
Pose 3 - Move legs only, knees locked.

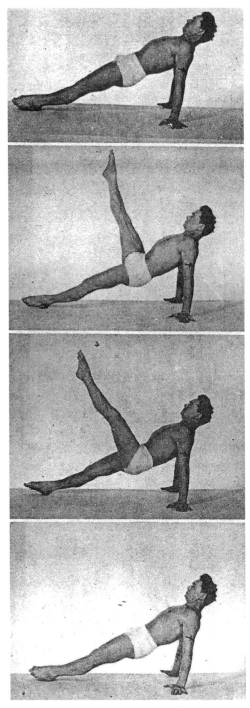

26. The Leg-Pull

INSTRUCTIONS for "The Leg-Pull"

Pose 1   (a) Take position illustrated
           (b) Arms (shoulder-wide) in right angle position
           (c) Hands at right angles
           (d) Head in straight line with body
           (e) Legs close together
           (f) Toes pointed downward
           (g) Heels close together
           (h) Knees locked

Pose 2   (a) INHALE SLOWLY
           (b) Raise right leg upward and backward as high as possible
           (c) EXHALE SLOWLY
           (d) Lower right leg to Pose 1 position

Pose 3   (a) INHALE SLOWLY
           (b) Raise left leg upward and backward as high as possible
           (c) EXHALE SLOWLY
           (d) Lower left leg to Pose 1 position

NOTE

Repeat the foregoing leg exercise three (3) times, right and left.

CAUTIONS

Pose 1 - Arms must be shoulder-wide in right angle position.
Pose 2 - Move legs only, knees locked.
Pose 3 - Move legs only, knees locked.

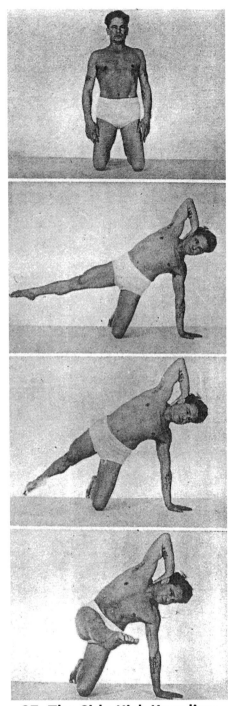

27. The Side Kick Kneeling

INSTRUCTIONS for "The Side Kick Kneeling"

Pose 1   (a) Take position illustrated

Pose 2   (a) Kneel on left knee and

            (b) Support body on left arm, then

            (c) Stretch right leg (knee locked) out sidewise in straight line with body

            (d) Toes (pointed) forward and downward, then

            (e) Bring right arm backward with hand supporting head, elbow back as far as possible, then

Pose 3   (a) INHALE QUICKLY while

            (b) "Swinging" right leg forward forcibly as far as possible,

Pose 4   (a) then EXHALE QUICKLY while

            (b) "Swinging" right leg backward forcibly as far as possible

Pose 2   (a) Kneel on right knee and

            (b) Support body on right arm, then

            (c) Stretch left leg (knee locked) out sidewise in straight line with body with

            (d) Toes (pointed) forward and downward, then

            (e) Bring left arm and elbow backward as far as possible with hand supporting head, then

Pose 3   (a) INHALE QUICKLY while

            (b) "Swinging" left leg backward forcibly as far as possible,

Pose 4   (a) then EXHALE QUICKLY while

            (b) "Swinging" left leg backward forcibly as far as possible

NOTE

Repeat the foregoing exercise four times with each leg.

CAUTIONS

Pose 2 - Keep head up, elbow back, chest out and abdomen in. Keep body rigid; move legs only. INHALE QUICKLY when swinging legs forcibly forward. EXHALE QUICKLY when swinging legs forcibly backward.

REMARKS

Concentrating on waistline and hips, also exercise for balance and coordination.

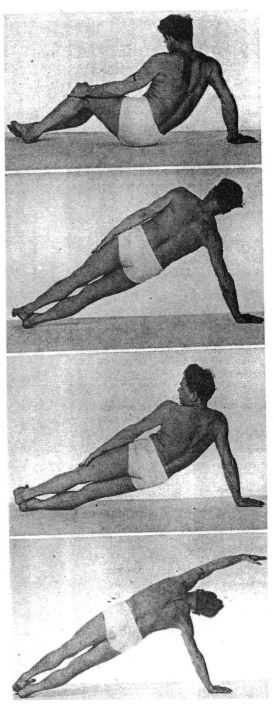

28. The Side Bend

INSTRUCTIONS for "The Side Bend"

Pose 1   (a) Take position illustrated

Pose 2   (a) Keep right arm in line with right shoulder
               (b) Left arm flat against body
               (c) Head up
               (d) Chin drawn in
               (e) Eyes straight forward
               (f) INHALE SLOWLY

Pose 3   (a) Turn head left and try to rest chin on left shoulder
               (b) Lower body until right calf touches mat or floor
               (c) EXHALE SLOWLY
               (d) Return to Pose 2 position
               (e) INHALE SLOWLY

NOTE

Repeat the foregoing exercise three (3) times, right and left.

CAUTIONS

Pose 2 - Keep body rigid, head up, chest out, abdomen "drawn" in.
Pose 3 - Only left and right calf respectively should touch mat when lowered.

REMARKS

This exercise concentrates on arm, shoulder and wrist muscles, stretches hip and waistline, and develops balance and coordination. Initially, you alternate between poses 2 and 3. After a month, begin to alternate between poses 4 and 2.

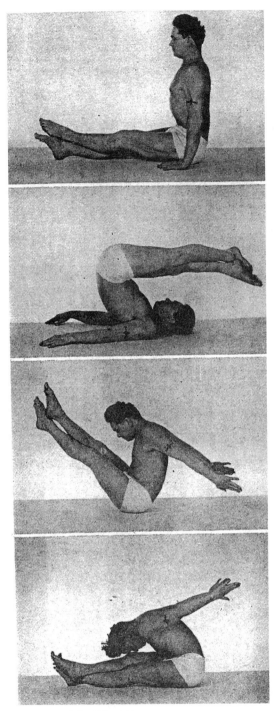

29. The Boomerang

INSTRUCTIONS for "The Boomerang"

Pose 1   (a) Take position illustrated
               (b) INHALE SLOWLY
               (c) Sit up straight in right angle position
               (d) Head up
               (e) Abdomen "drawn" in
               (f) Cross left leg over right leg
               (g) Arms pressed against body
               (h) Hands pointed forward and pressed against mat or floor

Pose 2   (a) EXHALE SLOWLY while
               (b) "Rolling" backward as far as possible and while in this position
               (c) Cross right leg over left leg and

Pose 3   (a) INHALE SLOWLY while
               (b) "Rolling" forward and
               (c) "Swing" arms backward as far as possible

Pose 4   (a) EXHALE SLOWLY while bringing both
               (b) Legs to mat or floor with
               (c) Head touching knees with
               (d) Arms (palms up) raised backward as far as possible and upward and
               (e) Return to Pose 2 position

NOTE

Repeat the foregoing exercise six (6) times, first starting with right leg crossed over left leg and then crossing left leg over right leg alternately.

CAUTIONS

Pose 2 - Keep arms and shoulders pressed firmly against mat or floor. Reverse legs while in "overhead" position when returning to Pose 3 position.

Pose 4 - Try to touch head to knees. Keep arms (palms up) stretched straight backward and upward as far as possible.

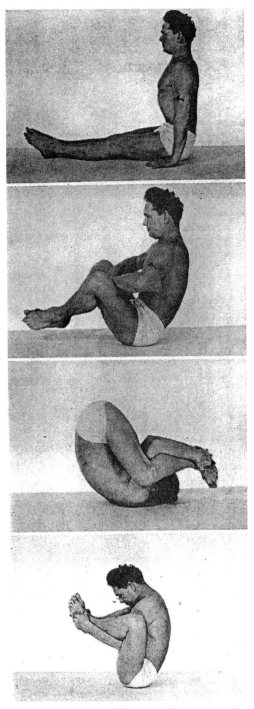

30. The Seal

INSTRUCTIONS for "The Seal"

Pose 1   (a) Take position illustrated

Pose 2   (a) INHALE SLOWLY
- (b) Bend head forward to chest
- (c) Abdomen pressed in
- (d) Legs apart "spread-eagle" fashion
- (e) Soles and heels together, pointed inward

Pose 3   (a) EXHALE SLOWLY
- (b) Twine both arms "grapevine" fashion under both legs
- (c) Passing left arm under and over left leg
- (d) Grasping left instep in locked grip
- (e) Passing right arm under and over right leg
- (f) Grasping right instep in locked grip
- (g) Press soles and heels firmly close together, pointed inward

Pose 4   (a) INHALE SLOWLY while
- (b) "Rolling" backward as far as possible
- (c) EXHALE SLOWLY
- (d) Return to Pose 3 position
- (e) "Clap" (hand-fashion) soles and heels together, twice

NOTE

Repeat the foregoing exercise six (6) times.

CAUTIONS

Pose 2 - Bend body forward. Press chest in. Tilt body backward to raise legs off mat or floor.

Pose 3 - "Pivot" body on rump in "rolling" backward and forward. You INHALE while "rolling" backward.

Pose 4 - Press head firmly to mat or floor in "rolling" upward. You EXHALE while "rolling" upward.

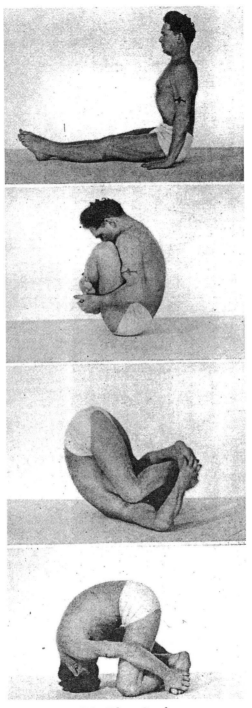

31. The Crab

INSTRUCTIONS for "The Crab"

Pose 1   (a) Take position illustrated
             (b) INHALE SLOWLY

Pose 2   (a) EXHALE SLOWLY
             (b) Cross legs Indian-fashion
             (c) Head bent forward
             (d) Chin to chest
             (e) Abdomen pressed in
             (f) Grasp both feet firmly
             (g) Right hand grasping left foot
             (h) Left hand grasping right foot
             (i) Pull" both knees toward shoulders as far as possible

Pose 3   (a) INHALE SLOWLY while
             (b) "Rolling" backward as far as possible
             (c) EXHALE SLOWLY while
             (d) "Rolling" upward until

Pose 4   (a) Head rests on mat or floor
             (b) INHALE SLOWLY until you return to Pose 3 position
             (c) EXHALE SLOWLY while again "rolling" upward until
             (d) Head rests on mat or floor as indicated in Pose 4

NOTE

Repeat the foregoing exercise six (6) times.

CAUTIONS

Pose 2 - Hold head as closely as possible to chest. Press abdomen in. "Round" back. "Pull" knees to shoulders as nearly as possible. "Pivot" on rump.

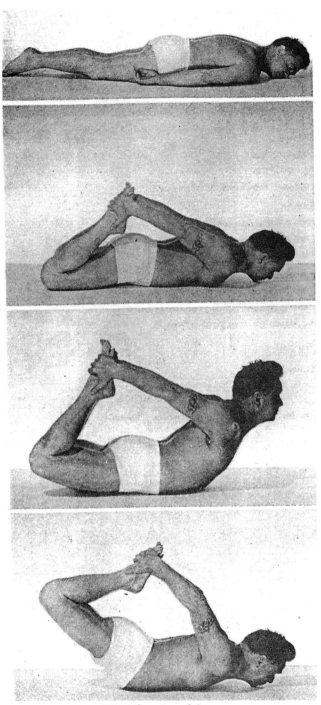

32. The Rocking

INSTRUCTIONS for "The Rocking"

Pose 1   (a) Take position illustrated
           (b) Rest body (face downward) on mat or floor
           (c) Press arms to sides with palms upward
           (d) Stretch legs (close together) backward
           (e) Keep toes (pointed) forward and downward

Pose 2   (a) Bend legs forward toward head
           (b) Grasp feet

Pose 3   (a) INHALE SLOWLY
           (b) Thrust chest out with head thrown back as far as possible
           (c) Stretch legs (close together) toward mat or floor

Pose 4   (a) Rock forward until chin touches mat or floor
           (b) Rock backward as far as possible
           (c) INHALE SLOWLY as you
           (d) Rock forward and
           (e) EXHALE SLOWLY as you
           (f) Rock backward

NOTE

Repeat the foregoing exercise five (5) times.

CAUTIONS

Pose 2 - Keep head thrown back as far as possible.

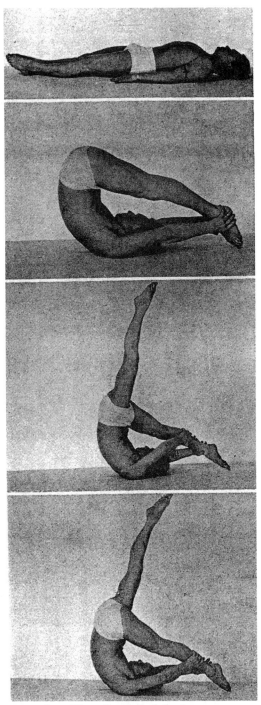

33. The Control Balance

INSTRUCTIONS for "The Control Balance"

Pose 1   (a) Take position illustrated
         (b) Rest entire body on mat or floor
         (c) Legs (close together) straight forward
         (d) Toes (pointed) forward and downward
         (e) Arms straight forward beside body
         (f) Palms down
         (g) INHALE SLOWLY
Pose 2   (a) EXHALE SLOWLY
         (b) "Roll" over until body rests on shoulders, arms and neck
Pose 3   (a) INHALE SLOWLY
         (b) Right toe touches mat or floor with
         (c) Right foot firmly grasped by both hands and
         (d) Left leg held straight upward as high as possible
Pose 4   (a) EXHALE SLOWLY
         (b) Release hold of hands on right foot and
         (c) Bring left leg downward until
         (d) Left toe touches mat or floor and
         (e) Grasp left foot firmly with both hands
         (f) Right leg held straight upward as high as possible

NOTE
Repeat Poses 3 and 4 of the foregoing exercise six (6) times.

CAUTIONS
Pose 2 Maintain balance on shoulders, arms and neck. Keep knees locked. Toes (pointed) forward and downward.

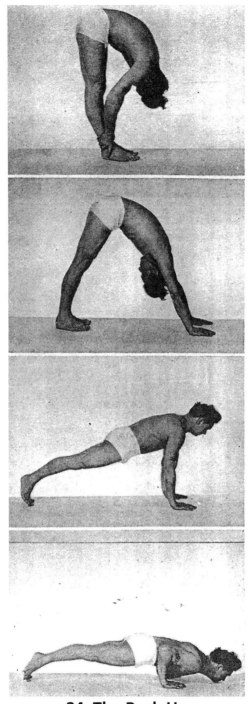

34. The Push Up

INSTRUCTIONS for "The Push Up"

Pose 1   (a) Take position illustrated
               (b) With arms (shoulder-wide) and palms extended
               (c) Try to touch mat or floor

Pose 2   (a) Keep feet pressed firmly on mat or floor
               (b) proceed "to walk" forward on palms of hands
               (c) Keep head downward and continue "walking" forward until

Pose 3   (a) You assume position illustrated in this pose
               (b) Keep body rigid and in a straight line from head to heels
               (c) Raise weight of body on toes and palms with
               (d) Arms (shoulder-wide) and hands pointed straight forward
               (e) Keep head in straight line with body

Pose 4   (a) Keep body rigid
               (b) Back locked
               (c) Bend arms (shoulder-wide) at elbows with
               (d) Upper arms pressed firmly to body
               (e) INHALE SLOWLY
               (f) Lower body until chin touches mat or floor
               (g) Stretch neck straight outward as far as possible
               (h) Hips locked
               (i) Abdomen "drawn" in
               (j) Chest raised above mat or floor
               (k) EXHALE SLOWLY
               (l) Raise body slowly by
               (m) Pressing hands firmly against mat or floor

NOTE

Repeat the foregoing exercise three (3) times.

CAUTIONS

Pose 3 - Keep shoulders in straight line with hands. Hips locked. Head in straight line with body. Keep body absolutely rigid. Move arms only (not body). Touch chin (not chest) to mat or floor.

Part III

21st Century Pilates Evolution

Table of Contents for Part III

21st Century Pilates Evolution

Introduction to Evolutionary Developments........................ 185

Pilates' Organizations:.. 190

Chapter 1: Pilates Magic Circle 191

Chapter 2: Weights.. 197

Chapter 3: Seated Pilates.. 203

Chapter 4: Mini Stability Ball 209

Chapter 5: Elastic Resistance 215

Chapter 6: Standing Work... 221

Chapter 7: Circular Work 227

Chapter 8: Unstable Surfaces 233

Chapter 9: Fusion Classes.. 239

Chapter 10: Sports Specific Pilates............................. 245

Appendix A: Glossary of Pilates' terms...................... 250

Appendix B: Index 254

Introduction to 21st Century Evolutionary Developments

Evolution, in the case of Pilates, began in 1934 with Your Health, continued in 1945 with Return to *Life through Contrology*, and continues to this very day with new exercises, new equipment, new enhancements to his original fitness programming, and *Pilates Evolution*.

Developments to and through the 21st Century

Pilates developed his fitness techniques in response to those that he himself experienced while growing up in Germany at the end of the 19th Century. At that time, many practitioners used specially invented apparatuses and claimed that what they offered could cure illness. As you've seen in Pilates' own writings, he quite strongly sided with this fundamental concept, although he also disagreed strongly with the specifics that others offered.

Pilates' first generation of students in New York, many of whom were dancers and choreographers, subsequently opened their own studios. They continued teaching Pilates' method with their own personal stamp; most became legends in the 20th Century, such as Romana Kryzanowska, Joe Grimes, Eve Gentry, and Ron Fletcher. More recent students of Pilates' methodologies, such as Moira Stott (now Stott-Merrithew) in Canada, Joan Breibart and Elizabeth Larkam in the US, have begun an irreversible evolutionary trend in the 21st Century world of Pilates' instruction.

While Pilates' original exercise systems focused on core strengthening with simultaneous spinal and limb stretching, STOTT PILATES aims in the 21st Century to offer a more progressive form of exercise, incorporating modern knowledge about the body and the more recent discoveries in exercise science and spinal rehabilitation. Stott's trainings have evolved to include more pelvic and shoulder girdle stabilization exercises, as well as emphasis on more anatomical concepts of neutral spine and pelvis. Moira herself studied and apprenticed with Romana Kryzanowska at the New York studio founded by Joseph Pilates.

Joan Breibart co-founded The Institute for the Pilates Method in Santa Fe, New Mexico in 1991, along with Michele Larsson and Eve Gentry. Although initially conceived of as an organization that would offer instructor training in Pilates' methods, it has since become quite innovative in expanding Pilates' methods with their own. Chapters 6 and 7 of this Part III focus on Standing Pilates® and Circular Pilates, two of Joan's primary evolutionary focuses. After moving her organization to New York City, and renaming it the PhysicalMind Institute, her organization continues to train thousands of current Pilates' instructors. Along with many others, she continues to enhance Pilates' work with modern awareness of biomechanical issues during vertical and horizontal exercises.

Elizabeth Larkam is a recognized innovator and developer of Pilates-based protocols for orthopedic, spinal and chronic pain diagnosis and treatment. She began her study of Pilates' techniques in 1985 while teaching dance at Stanford University and was another student of first generation Pilates' teachers Ron Fletcher, Eve Gentry and Romana Kryzanowska. A co-founder of Polestar Pilates Education, Elizabeth is a Master Teacher with Balanced Body University conducting courses throughout North America, Europe and Asia. Since 1992, Elizabeth has created dozens of instructional DVDs for fitness, therapeutic, education and home markets.

Another Master Teacher in Balanced Body University's programs is Madeline Black. Having worked with some of the greats in the Pilates and dance world --- Romana Kryzanowska, Eve Gentry, Marika Molnar and Irene Dowd --- she has herself become one of the 21st Century leaders in extending Joseph Pilates' legacy through her own innovative studies of movement. She specializes in integrating concepts and techniques, and evolving new methodologies and approaches, from Pilates, Gyrotonic®, yoga and other movement systems. The authors of this very book are very pleased to have received our certifications in Pilates from Madeline Black in 1993 when she was teaching for Joan Breibart's PhysicalMind Institute at her own San Francisco Studio M location (now in Sonoma County).

Elizabeth Larkam and Madeline Black are only two of the notable list of 21st Century stars in the evolutionary development of Pilates' based fitness education. Both of these women are Mentors in the Passing the Torch Program created by Balanced Body and themselves coach advanced teachers and trainers in the Pilates industry.

As program director of Balanced Body Pilates in Sacramento, California, Elizabeth developed instructional videos for their equipment, both large and small. Although the other notables mentioned above also work with companies that produce noteworthy Pilates' equipment, props, and training materials, Balanced Body deserves a special mention here, and not only because we ourselves have used and taught with Balanced Body equipment.

On October 19, 2000, Balanced Body and its founder/owner Ken Endelman won a U.S. Federal trademark lawsuit. Ken and his company were both sued by Sean Gallagher for trademark infringement, because Gallagher had purchased the trademark in 1992 and Ken among others was building and selling Pilates' inspired equipment. In short, the result of that lawsuit was that Pilates, like other generic fitness names such as karate or yoga, would no longer qualify for trademark infringement protection. Anyone from that moment on could use the name *Pilates* for the creation and offering of exercise services or equipment.

Evolutionary Props and Apparatus Developments

Romana Kryzanowska would correct interviewers when they asked her about Pilates' "machines". A "machine" does something to you, she would say, whereas with a Pilates' "apparatus", you are yourself guided to do the work and train your body. As you know, Pilate's original 34 mat exercises made no use of any apparatus or prop. Romana noted that if "you can do the mat work perfectly, you don't need the apparatus. But people love toys." As instructors, we have to agree, but they are more than simply entertainment; they are facilitators. The students must learn the exercises properly, with or without an apparatus or prop, in order to enable their body to reflect the intent of each exercise. As Pilates would say, people must "get the method in their bodies".

Each piece of apparatus or prop has a unique repertoire of exercises that have evolved from Pilates' principles that were seen earlier in this book. The most common large scale apparatus seen in traditional Pilates studios is the Reformer, although also seen are such imposing pieces as the Cadillac, special Chairs, and a variety of Barrels. As well, for both fun and body-targeted purposes, you can now see an explosion of new and increasingly used props, such as the Magic Circle, elastic tubes and straps, foam rollers, small and large exercise balls, weights, and other inventive devices that are introduced in the following chapters.

Classical Pilates' instructors often teach exercises in an unvarying order, staying close to Pilates' original work. Generally, they also use equipment that is built to his original specifications. Most classically trained teachers will have studied the complete system of exercises and can generally trace their training back to Joseph Pilates through one of his protégés. Contemporary/modern Pilates breaks the method down into various parts and the order of the exercises varies from lesson to lesson with many changes made to the original exercises.

Structure of each Chapter

Each of the upcoming ten chapters focuses on a different major area of Pilates' evolution, and does so in a consistent way. In the pages allotted to each subject, the first page introduces the technique or concept or prop or emphasis, while the chapter ends with a page devoted to resources from companies specializing in training, certification, videos or books. The remaining pages present new example exercises in the same manner that Pilates introduced his exercises a century ago.

We introduce at least two demonstrative exercises in each of the first nine chapters. Two facing pages include a series of photographs on the right side with step by step instructions on the left side. Visual sequencing allows you to use or teach a novel exercise that is both effective and fun. The instructions include explanations of the various aspects of the exercise, along with modifications for less or more advanced bodies.

Basic Pilates becomes even more challenging and more focused by using props and/or standing and moving variations. Adding exercise bands can offer increased resistance. Using foam rollers and other unstable objects can create stability challenges, and using props like the Magic Circle can offer additional options for strengthening legs and arms while simultaneously working core muscles. There is no required order to the following chapters. Feel free to jump to whichever interests you most; just be sure to go to the other chapters as well. They are all fun and innovative, and can help you strengthen your core while building balance, alleviating pain, and potentially rehabilitating from and reducing the likelihood of future injuries.

Pilates' Organizations: Certifications, Workshops & Products

Balanced Body®
>	http://www.pilates.com

BASI (Body Arts and Science International) Pilates®
>	http://www.basipilates.com/

Body Control Pilates
>	http://www.bodycontrol.co.uk

Michael Miller Pilates
>	http://www.hermit.com/

PeakPilates®
>	http://peakpilates.com/peak-pilates-home/

PhysicalMind Institute
>	http://themethodpilates.com/

Pilates Center of Boulder
>	http://www.thepilatescenter.com/

Pilates Institute of Australasia (Menezes Pilates)
>	http://www.pilates.net/

Pilates Method Alliance
>	http://www.pilatesmethodalliance.org/

Polestar Pilates
>	http://www.polestarpilates.com

STOTT PILATES®
>	http://www.stottpilates.com

United States Pilates Association® and the Pilates Guild™
>	http://www.unitedstatespilatesassociation.com/
>	http://www.pilates-studio.com/docs/guild/guild.htm

Chapter 1: Pilates Magic Circle

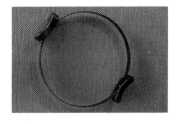

Romana Kryzanowska shares the entertaining story that Pilates got his original idea for the Magic Circle when he once removed a steel ring from a cognac keg. Inspired invention led to this flexible metallic or fiberglass ring with two cushioned handles on each side. The cushioning protects the hands, legs, or arms while holding it, as well as facilitating an even balance and alignment during exercises. At the same time, it enhances the core strengthening with the opportunity to tone the chest and upper body while strengthening the arms or legs. The Circle's flexibility provides variable resistance and results in enhanced awareness during exercises.

The Circle Facilitates Awareness

Resistance with a Circle is not aimed at bulking up muscles. Squeezing the Circle between legs or arms activates neuromuscular contraction and helps to sculpt your body and to develop a toned, conditioned physique without unduly increasing stress on your joints.

Proper Usage Leads to Effectiveness and Safety

Ensure that you've secured the Circle between arms or legs before squeezing it during an exercise. It should be evenly aligned, centered, and symmetrically balanced so as to minimize the possibility of it slipping out unexpectedly. Under compression from your limbs, it is possible that it could fly outwards and injure someone who is nearby.

During exercise in which your hands will be compressing the Circle, do not curl your fingers or tightly grip the Circle. Keep wrists straight and palms open and flat. Keep your fingers relaxed and elongated, using the heel of the hand to actually press inwards into the Circle. Finally, avoid excess tension in the joints by keeping your arms slightly rounded or knees slightly bent.

Core is Key

Regardless of where you position the Circle, and which additional muscles are targeted, remember that you should always concentrate first on the breath and the core muscles being activated. All movement begins from the core and moves outward from the 'powerhouse'.

Exercise #1: Chest Press

Stand relaxed, legs shoulder width apart, holding the Circle at chest height. Place the palm of each hand on the outer pads of the Circle, fingers extended. Inhale to begin. Exhale slowly to the count of four as you squeeze the Magic Circle, contracting your pectoral muscles. You can alternately perform the same exercise while lying on your back with knees bent and soles of the feet flat on the floor.

Exercise #2: Mid-Back

Follow the first exercise with a mid to upper back balancing exercise. Remain standing and bring the Circle around behind you, palms against the outer pads again. Inhale to begin. Exhale slowly to a count of four, as you squeeze the Magic Circle, engaging your back muscles and drawing your shoulder blades inward simultaneously. A seated version can be used as a modification. Follow the same instructions but bow forward from the hips for personal comfort or adjustment.

Exercise #3: Biceps

Use the same standing position as above. Place the Circle against your right shoulder. Bring your palm above the top pad and inhale to begin. As you exhale, push downwards toward the shoulder for a count of four. Inhale to relax, and repeat. After the standard number of repetitions, switch to the left shoulder.

Exercise #4: Lat Press

Place the Magic Circle horizontally against your hip. Place your palm against the Circle, fingers extended. Inhale to begin. Exhale to a count of four as you squeeze the Circle inward against your body. Repeat eight times on one side, and then repeat on the other side.

Tips

The slow exhalations cued above can be changed to a rapid series of exhalation puffs instead. Also, when lifting the Magic Circle, be sure to keep your shoulders down and relaxed. Imagine that you are drawing your shoulder blades downward.

Repetitions

Repeat eight times per exercise before moving on to the next variation. As you become stronger, you can increase the repetitions from eight to ten or twelve.

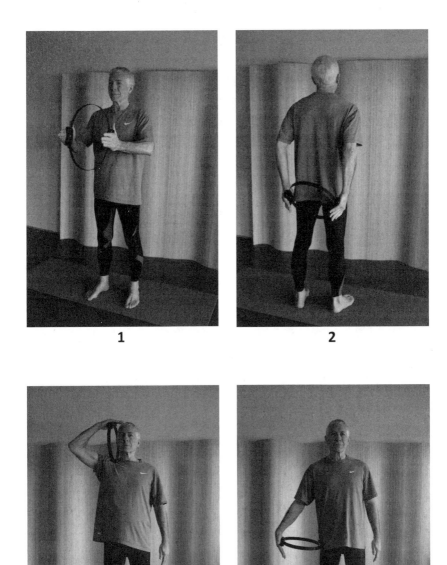

1

2

3

4

Exercises #1 - 4 (Magic Circle)

Pose #1: One leg braces the ring; other leg prepares to move

- Lie on your right side lengthwise, supporting your upper body with both arms stabilizing you. Place the ankle of your right leg just inside the Magic Circle, bracing it against the ground in a vertical position.
- If this positioning is uncomfortable for your back, you can adjust your straight legs slightly forward into an overall body banana position. This will be more stabilizing and protect your back a bit more.
- Extend your left leg outside the Circle, toes pointed close to the floor in front. Inhale to begin.

Pose #2: Exhaling to begin to trace the rainbow

Slowly exhale to begin arcing your extended left leg upwards along the outside of the Circle.

Pose #3: Slow, continuous exhalation during the rainbow

Continue exhaling and tracing a rainbow path along the outside top of the Circle until your left leg reaches the floor at the rear of the Circle.

Pose #4: Inhaling to reverse back to the beginning

Reverse the rainbow path while inhaling and returning the leg.

Tips

In pose #1, you could alternatively relieve possible tension by placing your right elbow on the ground, and support your head with your right hand. Even further, you could rest your head against your entire outstretched right arm along the floor.

Repetitions

- Repeat six times per exercise before moving on to the next variation. As you become stronger, you can increase the repetitions from six to eight or ten.
- After finishing the repetitions on the right side, switch to your left side, reversing all instructions above. The left leg now braces the Circle, while the right leg traces the rainbow during the breath cycles.
- Beginners could trace a smaller path by placing the moving leg inside the Circle.

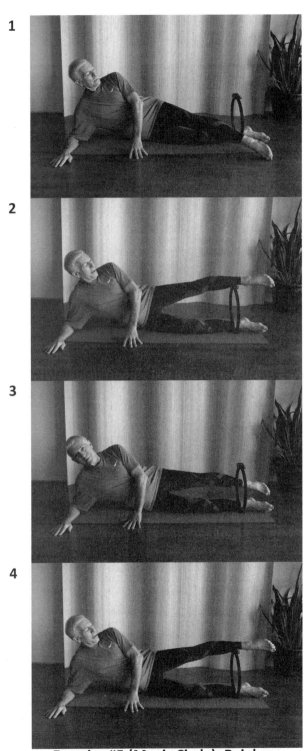

Exercise #5 (Magic Circle): Rainbow

BOOKs

Ellie Herman's Pilates Props Workbook: Illustrated Step-by-Step Guide
　　　　By Ellie Herman

DVDs

STOTT PILATES: Fitness Circle Flow
　　　　With Moira Merrithew and Wayne Seeto

Winsor Pilates 20 Minute Circle Workout
　　　　by Guthy - Renker

Winsor Pilates Sculpting Circle (Beginner & Advanced DVDs)
　　　　From Winsor Pilates

West Coast Pilates Magic Circle for Body Balance Work-out
　　　　From West Coast Pilates

Classical Pilates Technique: The Complete Magic Circle Matwork Series
　　　　By Bob Liekens

BOOK & DVD

Pilates with Workout Circle Book & DVD Box Set
　　　　by Dina Matty

MAGIC CIRCLE & DVD

Stamina Pilates Magic Circle with Workout DVD
　　　　From Stamina

MP4 Downloadable Videos (3 levels)

Look up "Magic Circle"
　　　　At http://www.iAmplify.com

Chapter 2: Weights

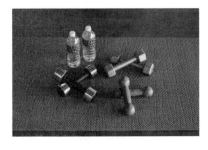 Light hand weights are inexpensive commonplace, and easy to use. You could also replace hand weights with wrist weights in Pilates' exercises and variations. This may be advisable if you have any issues with wrist strength.

Let Caution Be Your Guide

Regardless of which type of weights you choose to employ in your exercises, keep in mind the fundamental focus of your attention during Pilates' work should be to work from the core outwards to the extremities. Using light weights can add an extra measure of stabilization for your shoulders, core and pelvis. Obviously, the amount of weight depends on your body size and current strength levels. A rough guide might be one to five (1–5) pound weights. Anything heavier can cause alignment problems, which would be completely counter to one of the primary goals of Pilates work. Heavy weights can not only pull you out of alignment, but they can place undue stress on your neck and shoulders or back and legs. Your focus can easily shift, with reduced benefits and increased dangers, from core to extremities.

Additional Benefits

Using lighter weights allows us to add a controlled amount of extra muscle toning to each exercise. Careful attention to the weights enables you to extend from the core out through your chest, shoulders, back and arms, or down through your hips and legs. Remember that Pilates' exercises should be practiced in concert with the breath work, with a maintained concentration during both phases of the breath, and during both concentric and eccentric contractions of the core muscles. Light weights add a little challenge while facilitating extra attention during the entire movement.

Do not use heavy weights simply because you mistakenly may see them as an opportunity to expend more energy and possibly lose weight. Weight loss or cardio benefits should be secondary to fundamental Pilates' principles.

Instructions for Double Leg Stretch w/Biceps Curls

Pose #1: Tabletop to begin

Begin by lying on your back with a relaxed, neutral spine. Knees are raised and bent with shins and feet forward in tabletop position. Arms are relaxed on the floor, with each hand holding a weight. Palms begin facing upwards but resting on the floor. Inhale to begin.

Pose #2: Bicep curl w/lifted vertical legs

Slowly exhale while:

- lifting your legs straight upwards, keeping your tailbone against the mat
- lifting your head and shoulders off the mat
- looking forwards towards your legs
- lifting the hands and weights toward you, keeping elbows on the mat

Pose #3: Double leg stretch, reversing the bicep curl

Slowly inhale while:

- lowering your legs to (at most) a 45° angle.
- keeping your low back pressed against the mat
- lowering the weights and hands back to their starting position

Continuing: Repeat Poses 2 and 3 the desired number of times

When you have finished the set (the desired number of repetitions, as below), simply draw your knees inward toward your chest, lower your head and shoulders, and finally lower the legs to the floor.

Tips

- If your neck feels strained during the repetitions of this combination sequence, you can focus on the legs and arms only by leaving your head and shoulders resting on the mat, as in pose #1. Save the head and shoulders lift for a future more challenging variation.
- If you are traveling or find yourself somewhere without weights, you can substitute a pair of water bottles.

Repetitions

Repeat four times as a set before taking a break, or moving on to another exercise. As you become stronger, you can increase the repetitions from four to six or eight.

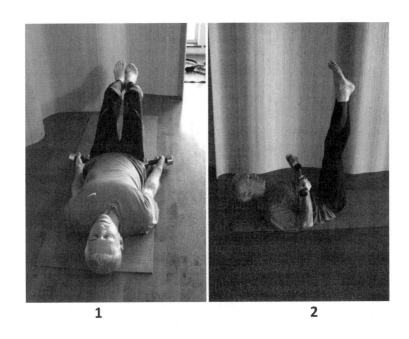

1   2

3

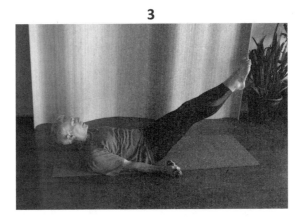

Exercise #6 (Weights): Double Leg Stretch w/Biceps Curls

Instructions for Front Shoulder Bridge with Weights

Pose #1: Arms raised to begin

Lie on your back with your knees up, soles of your feet on the ground. Inhale while lifting hands and weights straight upwards. Keep your shoulders relaxed and in contact with the mat.

Pose #2: Lift to bridge to continue

Exhale while lifting your hips upwards to a bridge pose.

Pose #3: Opening arms outward

Retain the bridge pose. Inhale while lowering your arms outwards and downwards.

Transition for Repetitions: Lowering hips to complete

Slowly exhale while rolling your spine downward to the mat. Repeat the entire sequence of poses 1 to 3 the desired number of repetitions.

Tips

In pose 2 and the transition back to pose 1, while slowly exhaling, you should have a sense of peeling your spine off the ground, or lowering it back to the ground, one vertebra at a time, as you create or reverse the bridge position.

Repetitions

Repeat six times per complete exercise. As you become stronger, you can increase the repetitions from six to eight or ten.

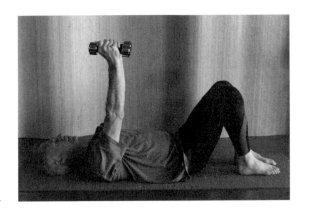

1

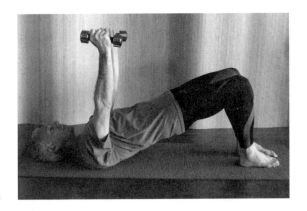

2

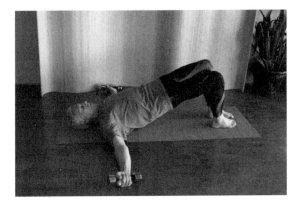

3

Exercise #7 (Weights): Front Shoulder Bridge

Resources

BOOKs

101 Ways to Work Out with Weights: Effective Exercises to Sculpt Your Body and Burn Fat!

    By Cindy Whitmarsh

DVDs

Senior Easy Light Weights Exercise DVD: Seniors / Elderly

    By Sunshine

DVD Kick Butt! WHFN FitPrime PUSH PULL Pilates Yoga Weights

    By Heidi Tanner and Kimberly Spreen

Sexy Body Workout - Pilates with Weights

    By Jonathan Urla and Christina Orloff

Golden Earth Pilates Yoga Wrist Weight Workout DVD

    From Golden Earth

The Authentic Complete Pilates Arm Series w/wo weight + Magic Circle Series; Stdg/Sitting/Lying + The Wall + Pilates Key Principals

    By Catherine Isaacson

WEIGHTs & DVD

Gaiam Mari Winsor's Pilates Bootcamp Kit

    From Gaiam

Chapter 3: Seated Pilates

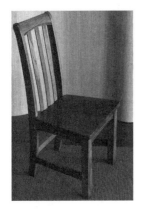

Although many of Pilates' original exercises, like Spine Stretch and Saw, were performed in a 'seated' position on the floor, this chapter concentrates on enhancements to Pilates' exercises while seated in a chair. A great deal of epidemiological research substantiates that many of our musculoskeletal disorders are directly attributable to overexertion or repetitive motion injuries, many of which occur while seated.

Benefits of Seated Pilates

Many of us spend enormous hours each day at a desk or in front of a computer, and opportunities abound for short breaks with easy Pilates' exercises while still in those chairs. Seated Pilates' exercises can also be extremely beneficial for individuals who suffer from limited mobility. Besides offering an easy approach to increasing strength and flexibility throughout your entire body, Pilates' exercises while seated can tone your abs, legs & glutes without even leaving the chair.

Basic Seated Guidelines

In all chair exercises, you should start with your feet flat on the ground, your lower legs and knees at right angles, your back straight and lengthened upwards, and your shoulders and arms drawn lightly back. During each exercise, strive to coordinate your (full) exhalations with the exertion phase of the exercise, and your (full) inhalations with the release or relaxation phase. Please sit all the way back into your chair, rather than perched near the front of it. Remember also to balance your shoulders over your center and balance your hips as well.

Seated Pilates is for Professionals of any Age or Fitness Level

Pilates' professionals often emphasize the value of Pilates work as it translates into daily life activities. Seated Pilates is not simply for seniors or those with decreased mobility. Many people with no seeming mobility problems suffer from back, neck and shoulder pain and do not realize that Pilates work in all its forms can improve posture and balance muscles, ligaments, tendons, and joints as a result.

Instructions for the Seated Pilates 100s

Pose #1: Seated without strap

- Sit on a chair with your feet flat on the ground and your knees bent at right angles over the front of the chair.
- Sit fully into the chair rather than on the front edge of the chair.
- Draw your shoulder blades gently downwards. Press your arms into extension while pulling your shoulders together.
- Pay attention to a balance between your shoulders, both left to right, and centered over your hips.
- All breaths should be slow and continuous, smoothly transitioning between inhales and exhales.
- Repeat the presses of the hands 100 times (See **Repetitions** section below for a detailed explanation).

Pose #2: Seated without strap, but with single leg extensions

This is similar to pose 1, except that you will extend one leg for the first fifty presses of the hands (five complete breath cycles). Then, lower that leg and raise the other leg for the second 50 presses of the hands.

Pose #3: Seated with strap in front

Using a strap or a tube for extra challenge and resistance, you would place the center of the strap across your midsection (or across the front of your legs) and hold or clasp the resistance at each end. With palms facing backwards, begin the 100 by pressing backwards.

Pose #4: Seated with strap in rear

Similar to pose 3, place the strap or tube behind the back. Clasp or hold it with palms facing forwards while completing the 100.

Tips

You can also sit on the ground cross-legged or with legs straight in front of you. Slightly angling your arms outwards will allow you to perform the 100 exercise without hitting the floor with your hands.

Repetitions

100 total presses, consisting of ten complete breath cycles. Each breath cycle in the traditional Pilates' 100 contains five presses per inhalation and five presses per exhalation. Each set of ten presses represents a breath cycle, and ten breath cycles in total represents the traditional warm up exercise, the Pilates' 100.

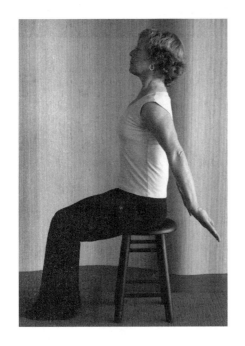

1

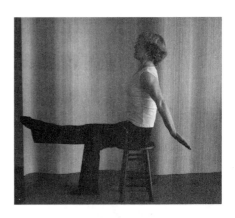

2

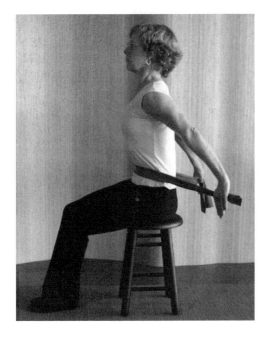

3

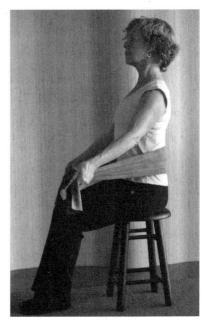

4

Exercise #8 (Seated Pilates): Seated 100's

Instructions for the Seated Swan

Pose #1: Starting position
- Rest your hands on your thighs.
- Slowly exhale while lowering your chin and eyes to gaze at your hands.

Pose #2: Pressing into extension
- Slowly inhale while raising your chin and head, but do not allow your gaze to rise above the horizontal.
- Press downwards with your hands into your thighs.
- Continue to gaze straight ahead while continuing to lift your head.
- Simultaneously, lengthen your back while gently arching your spine.

Pose #3: Rounding forward
- Slowly exhale while lifting your hands upwards to chest height.
- Lower your eyes to gaze directly at your hands.
- Simultaneously, allow your back, spine, and elbows to round.

Pose #4: Pressing backwards into 2nd extension
- Slowly inhale while lowering and straightening your arms.
- Press your arms directly backwards and slightly outwards while raising your eyes to look directly forward again.

Tips
Be careful not to force your spine into any position. Allow your back to lengthen and extend gracefully, without forcing it into any excessive curvature.

Repetitions
Repeat four times per complete exercise. As you become stronger, you can increase the repetitions from six to eight.

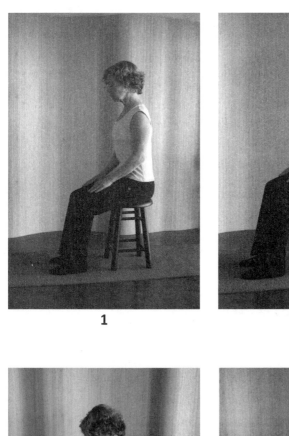

1

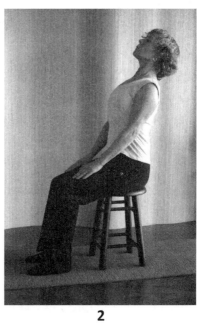

2

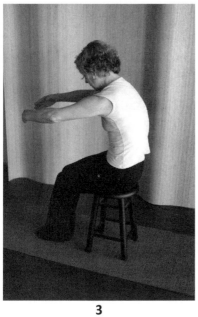

3

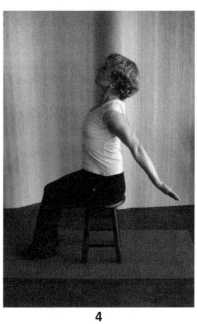

4

Exercise #9 (Seated Pilates): Seated Swan

Resources

BOOKs

Mind Your Body: Pilates for the Seated Professional
  By Juli Kagan

DVDs

Stronger Seniors® Core Fitness: Chair-based Pilates
  By Anne Pringle Burnell

Stronger Seniors® Chair Exercise Program- 2 disc Chair Exercise Program
  By Anne Pringle Burnell

Susan Tuttle's In Home Fitness: Chair Pilates
  By Susan Tuttle

Chair Pilates with Nikki Carrion
  by FitXpress .com

Seniors Exercise DVD: Senior / Elderly Sitting Exercises
  By Sunshine

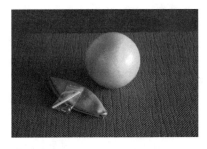

We first became aware of the soft mini ball for Pilates' exercises when Leslee Bender in Nevada released the Bender Method of Core Training with a 9" stability ball known then and now as a Bender ball. We have enjoyed the creativity seen in her program as have our students. Many exercises with larger exercise balls can easily be modified to use this smaller size. This in turn offers opportunities to instructors for creative enhancements to programming.

In many cases, the mini balls prove easier for students to manipulate (not to mention being easier to store and transport) than the larger stability balls. A variety of competitive companies now offer similar type small balls. Be sure to avoid overinflating your mini ball to decrease likelihood of breakage and to retain the flexibility benefits.

Benefits of a Mini Ball Pilates' Workout

Using the small ball can reduce strain on back muscles while strengthening overall core muscles. Bender's concept aims to relax what is tight, and strengthen what is weak. The ball can support the back while also strengthening the core muscles.

A Range of Pilates Benefits

A consistent element of many mini ball exercises is the squeezing of the ball with either hands or legs. This facilitates strengthening chest, shoulders, arms and legs while focusing on the core muscles. Placement of the ball itself allows a wide range of fun variations. For example, you can focus on your abdomen by holding the mini ball directly in front of your stomach while squeezing it and tightening your buttocks. The mini ball can equally well complement other evolutionary techniques like standing work or seated work for postural gains and leg strengthening.

A Few Cautions Are in Order

Although a mini-ball workout is quite fun, many of the exercises target core muscles through balance. Anyone suffering from any sort of balance difficulties should take extra care when following any mini-ball exercises.

Pose #1: Starting position

Lie back on the mat with knees bent and legs comfortably in line with shoulders and hips. Take the mini ball between your hands and extend your arms overhead to approximately ear height. Do not arch your back. Inhale to begin.

Pose #2: Round up with ball

Slowly exhale to a count of four as you lift your head and round your back and shoulders upwards. Draw your belly downwards, hollowing your abdomen as your bottom ribs fold towards your hip bones. Reach your arms and ball forwards, placing the ball between your knees.

Pose #3: Reset arms

Slowly inhale to a count of four, drawing your ribs away from the hips, lowering your spine, vertebra by vertebra, as you extend your arms upwards toward your ears. Squeeze the ball between your knees as you descend towards the mat.

Pose #4: Lift to bridge

Slowly exhale to a count of four, contracting your gluteal muscles while lifting your hips upwards. Avoid any tension in your chest and evenly distribute the weight across your shoulders. Continue to squeeze the ball with your knees.

Transition from pose 4 back to pose 1 by:

- inhaling slowly to another count of four while lowering your hips to the mat.
- exhaling to a count of four while rounding your torso and head back up to take the ball back into your hands.
- inhaling to a count of four while lowering your arms, head and shoulders back to pose 1 above. Be careful to maintain the same separation between your knees at all times.

Tips

In poses 2 and 4, concentrate on the spinal flexion during rounding. Avoid any inclination to round or tense the shoulders.

Repetitions

Repeat eight times per exercise before moving on to the next variation. As you become stronger, you can increase the repetitions from eight to ten or twelve.

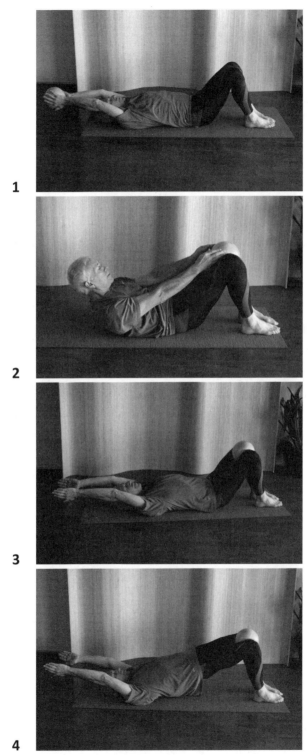

1

2

3

4

Exercise #10 (Mini Stability Ball): Shoulder Bridge Combo w/Ball

Instructions for Oblique Criss-Cross

Pose #1: Starting position

Lie on your back with both legs in tabletop position. Place the mini ball against your thighs just above the knees. Place your hands behind your head and lock the ball into position by drawing your elbows up against the ball. Inhale to begin.

Pose #2: First side position

Slowly exhaling to a count of four, draw your left elbow backwards and extend your right leg forwards. Hold the ball in place by squeezing it with your right elbow and left leg. Extending the leg up at an angle is less challenging than lengthening it straight forwards, parallel to the ground. Allow your head and torso to twist gently during the exhalation and rotation.

Pose #3: Transfer mid position

Slowly inhale to a count of four while returning your left elbow and right leg back to the starting position seen in pose 1 above.

Pose #4: Second side position

Reverse to the other side by slowly exhaling to a count of four, drawing your right elbow backwards and extending your left leg forwards. Hold the ball in place by squeezing it with your left elbow and right leg. Choose once again whether to extend this leg up at an angle, or, alternately, take the more challenging option of lengthening it straight forwards, parallel to the ground. Allow your head and torso to twist gently during the exhalation and rotation. Begin a new repetition by slowing inhaling to a count of four while returning arm and leg to pose 1.

Tips

Gain a more consistent and deeper involvement of the oblique abdominals by keeping each movement smooth and flowing with the breath. Do not hold your breath at any point, even during transfer of the ball from side to side.

Repetitions

Repeat eight times per complete breath cycle. As you become stronger, you can increase the repetitions from eight to ten or twelve.

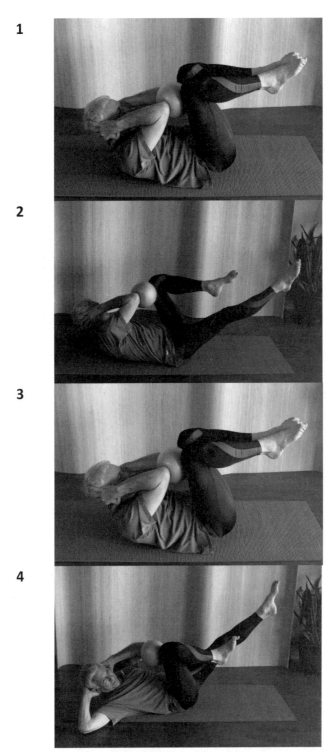

Exercise #11 (Mini Stability Ball): Oblique Criss-Cross

BOOKs

Franklin Method Ball and Imagery
> By Eric Franklin

DVDs

Bender Ball: The Bender Ball Method of Pilates Evolution
> From Bender Ball

Pilates Mini-Ball Advanced Workout
> By Leslee Bender

Pilates: Miniball
> By Juliana Afram

10 Minute Solution: Quick Sculpt Pilates with Toning Ball
> By Andrea Leigh Rogers

Pilates on the Go - Strengthen Your ABS & Back, Improve your Posture
> By Michaela Sirbu

STOTT PILATES: Mini Flex-Ball Workout
> By Moira Merrithew

BALL & DVD

Element Total Body Pilates With Mini Ball Kit
> With Lisa Hubbard

Gaiam Pilates Body Sculpting Workout Kit: 6" Pilates Ball & DVD
> From Gaiam

Stott Pilates Mini Stability-Ball Power Pack
> By Stott Pilates

Chapter 5: Elastic Resistance

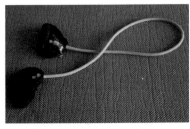 Elastic resistance bands or tubes are very common props in Pilates' studios, clubs, and classes. Inexpensive and easy to store, you can actually speed up development and reduce some discomfort in certain exercises while you train your body in both strength and flexibility. A number of simple exercises have evolved with bands or tubes by replicating other exercises seen earlier with a large scale (and expensive) Pilates Reformer. Often, one can logically substitute the band or tube for the spring tension on the larger piece of equipment.

Some Usage Guidelines

Resistance bands or tubes can add a varying amount of resistance to a Pilates' exercise by wrapping the elastic an extra time or two around your hands or feet. Creative design of exercises can generate interest and fun during your workout. Putting these techniques together achieves multiple benefits including lengthening and strengthening targeted muscles, and enhancing focus, concentration and exercise flow.

In lying, sitting, and standing positions, elastic resistance is commonly employed by wrapping the center of the tube/band around your feet, or simply stepping or sitting on it to fix its position. Once stabilized, and while holding the other ends, the body can be moved in a variety of ways. Standard Pilates' exercises become more challenging, and easily adjustable, according to where you place your hands on the tube/band.

A Few Tips and Cautions

A new student should first master a movement without elastic resistance. Add resistance to an exercise only after you've learned the elements of the movement and have developed enough strength to warrant adding the extra challenge. A subtle benefit of using resistance bands is that they can help you to deepen a stretch and focus your body movements on core strengthening elsewhere in the body (for example, during a rollup using a tube or strap around the legs).

Instructions for Lunging Biceps/Triceps

Pose #1: Starting prep position for biceps curls

From a standing position, step the right leg forward into a lunge position toward the front edge of the mat. Draw the left leg backwards, or angle the rear foot outwards for balance (about 30 degrees). Place the center of the tube underneath the arch of the forward right foot, holding onto the ends of the elastic with your hands. Inhale to a count of two.

Pose #2: Actual curl movement

Exhale to a count of two to pull your hands and the elastic resistance upwards toward your shoulders, bending the elbows as much as possible and keeping the upper arms tucked against your ribs. Inhale to lower the hands downwards back to pose 1, and repeat poses 1 and 2 the desired number of repetitions. Then switch legs and repeat.

Pose #3: Starting prep position for lunging triceps

From a standing position, step the right leg forward into a lunge position toward the front edge of the mat. Angle the rear left leg outwards for balance, just about 30 degrees. Place the center of the tube or strap underneath the arch of the forward right foot, holding onto the ends of the elastic resistance with your hands. Bow your torso forward from the hips to line your spine up with your rear left leg. Lift your elbows upwards behind you, inhaling for a count of two to begin.

Pose #4: Actual lunging triceps

Exhale to a count of two to pull your hands and the elastic resistance backwards behind you, straightening the elbows and arms. Keep the upper arms close to your ribs. Inhale to lower the hands downwards back to pose 3, and repeat poses 3 and 4 the desired number of repetitions. Then switch legs, stepping the left leg forward and repeat.

Tips

For more of a challenge in exercises 12 or 13, you could inhale and exhale to counts of one rather than two. Also, if angling the rear leg outwards for 30 degrees is difficult for your ankles, you could step the rear leg backwards, raising the heel for an alternate form of balance.

Repetitions

Repeat eight times with one leg forward before switching to the other leg. As you strengthen, increase repetitions from eight to ten or twelve.

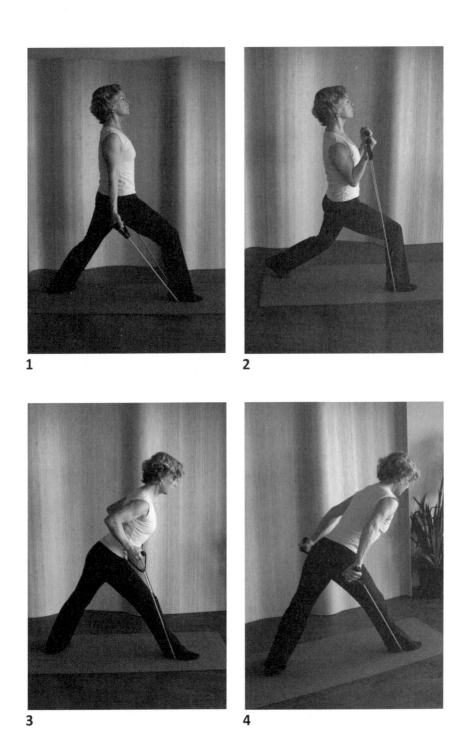

Exercise #12-13 (Elastic Resistance): Lunging Biceps/Triceps

Pose #1: Starting position

Lie on your back with legs together in tabletop position. Wrap the strap or tube around the soles of your feet. Draw the elastic resistance towards you, placing your upper arms against the mat. Inhale to begin.

Pose #2: Rolling up to prepare

Slowly exhale to a count of four as you lift your head and round your back and shoulders upwards. Draw your belly downwards, hollowing your abdomen as your bottom ribs fold toward your hip bones.

Pose #3: Pressing

Keeping your elbows firmly planted against the mat; continue exhaling to another count of four as you extend your legs. The angle that your legs make with the floor determines how challenging the press will be. Pressing the legs forward while remaining close to the floor will be the most challenging. Angling them upwards will be easier. Allow your forearms to align with the angle of the legs.

Pose #4: Lifting

Slowly inhale to a count of four as you straighten the legs upwards to a 90 degree angle. Finish the inhale while returning to pose 1 and repeat for the desired number of overall repetitions.

Tips

If a count of four is too long in both exhalation phases of poses 2 and 3, you can reduce the breathing count to two. If you want additional challenge, you can extend the count in poses 2 and 3 to counts of four as you roll up, and another four as you extend the legs.

Repetitions

Repeat eight times per exercise before moving on to the next variation. As you become stronger, you can increase the repetitions from eight to ten or twelve.

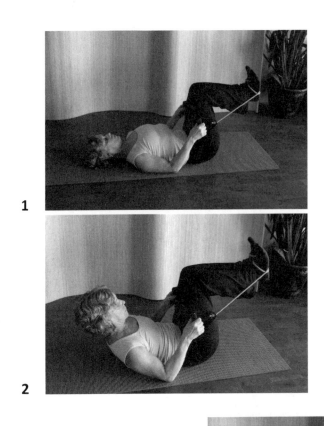

1

2

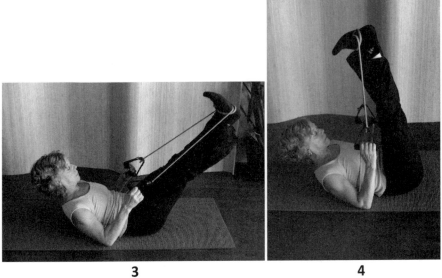

3

4

Exercise #14 (Elastic Resistance): Press-Lift Combo

Resources

BOOKs

Ellie Herman's Pilates Props Workbook: Illustrated Step-by-Step Guide
>   By Ellie Herman

The Resistance Band Workout Book [Paperback]
>   By Ed Mcneely and David Sandler

Sanctband Pilates Essentials [Paperback]
>   By Angela Kneale

DVDs

Winsor Pilates: Power Sculpting with Resistance (Multiple DVDs)
>   By Mari Winsor

Stott Pilates: Intense Sculpting Challenge
>   By Moira Merrithew

Pilates Bodyband Challenge
>   By Ana Caban

West Coast Pilates CORE Band™ Workouts (3 Levels Available)
>   From West Coast Pilates

Senior, Elderly Sitting Chair Pilate's Exercise DVD with Resistance Bands
>   By Sunshine

DVD & BANDs

Stott Pilates Flex-Band Kit
>   By Stott Pilates

The FIRM Sculpt and Tone Pilates
>   By The Firm

Chapter 6: Standing Work

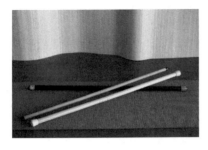

Ron Fletcher is internationally well known for his many contributions to Pilates' evolution over the last century. He was one of the first to bring Pilates' exercise off the mat and into standing positions. In clinical settings, assessment of postural problems is typically diagnosed in a standing position. Fletcher used visual cues to place emphasis on core posture during daily activities. The Fletcher Standing and Centering™ cues continue to underlie his popular and effective standing program.

Fletcher as 20th Century Innovator

As with other evolutionary teachers of renown, his work integrates basic Pilates' tenets with more current anatomical and physiological teachings that incorporate foot placement and articulation, bilateral symmetry both in stasis and in movement, dynamic pelvic stabilization, and spatial awareness during directional and level changes. His other evolutionary developments include the unique Fletcher Towelwork® program that literally uses a rolled up towel, for which one could easily substitute a bar, a stick, or even a mini-ball. His wide ranging syllabus spans a full repertoire from simple range of motion exercises to challenging and complex shoulder girdle, chest, head and spine movements.

Breibart & PhysicalMind Institute - 20th/21st Century Innovators

In 1991 Joan Breibart co-founded The Institute for the Pilates Method in Santa Fe, New Mexico along with Michele Larsson and Eve Gentry, one of the original Pilates elders. Known today as The PhysicalMind Institute, it has trained thousands of instructors and continues training Pilates' professionals as well as providing continuing education for its members. Her standing work is a natural evolution to the vertical position, like Fletcher's, and she continues to evolve her own trainings. She introduced a more energetic and engaging series of standing exercises with the Tye4, a neoprene mini-vest with bungee cording that attaches to the hands and feet. This adds resistance and new options for her Standing Pilates® repertoire.

Instructions for Chest Expansion

Pose #1: Starting position

Stand in a relaxed pose with feet hip width apart. Shoulders are relaxed, and arms are relaxed downwards.

Pose #2: Pressing backwards

Slowly inhale to a count of four while rising off the heels of both feet and pressing your arms backwards.

Pose #3: Turning the head in one direction

While holding your breath, and staying up on the balls of your feet, slowly turn your head to one direction.

Pose #4: Turning the head in other direction

Continue holding your breath while turning your head to the other direction.

End this pose exhaling slowly to a count of four while returning your head to the center and lowering down to the starting position of pose 1 above. Repeat the desired number of repetitions.

Tips

As you rise up, and while you are holding that position, stay centered over your feet and balanced from left to right. A slight emphasis toward the inside edges of the balls of your feet will aid in maintaining a vertical lift and balance.

Repetitions

Repeat six times per exercise before moving on to the next variation. As you become stronger, you can increase the repetitions from six to eight or ten.

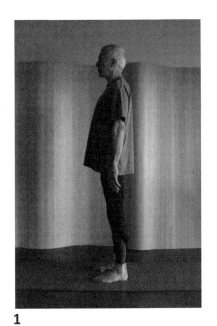
1

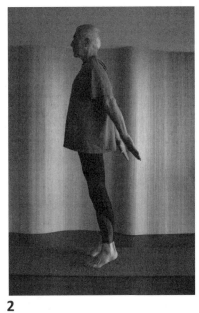
2

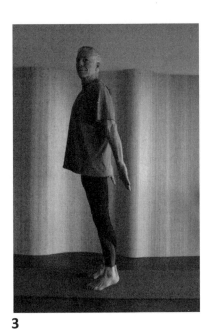
3

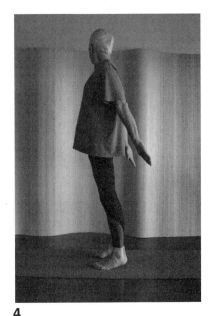
4

Exercise #15 (Standing Pilates): Chest Expansion

Preparing for the Complete Exercise

Stand in a relaxed, balanced pose with legs hip width apart. Using a stick or cane or pole or bar as an aid to holding a balance during all of these poses is a ready option, and is displayed in the pictures. Following the instructions without a balancing aid is just a little more challenging.

Pose #1: Abductor opening

Slowly inhale to a count of four while lifting your right leg out to the right side, keeping the kneecap facing forward. Have the feeling of lengthening upwards through your entire body while inhaling.

Pose #2: Adductor cross over

Slowly exhale to a count of four, while crossing your right leg in front of you (toward the balancing pole, if you are using one) and leading with your heel.

Pose #3: Front leg lift/flexion

Begin to inhale for a count of one while releasing your right leg back to center. Continue to inhale for another three counts while lifting it forward away from the body.

Pose #4: Back leg lift/extension

Slowly exhale for a count of four while extending the straight right leg backwards, either maintaining it in a straight form or bending it at the knee behind you into a dancer's 'attitude' pose. End this pose and the entire 4-way leg flow exercise by relaxing the leg back to the preparatory starting position. A continuous, flowing exercise movement would have you inhaling out of pose 4, as you lower the leg down, and flowing directly into the inhalation cued above as moving into pose 1.

Tips

As with all Pilates' exercise, try to engage in smooth, flowing movements in all four directions. Move your legs in concert with the flow of your breath.

Repetitions

Repeat eight times with one leg before moving on to the same exercise for another eight repetitions with the other leg. As you become stronger, you can increase the repetitions from eight to ten or twelve.

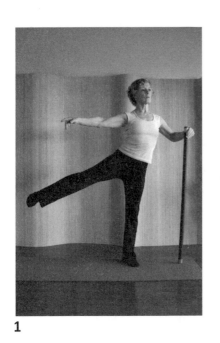

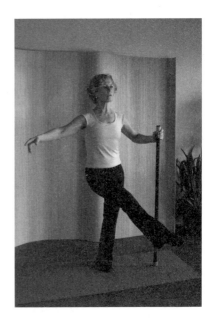

1

2

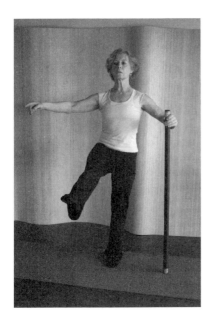

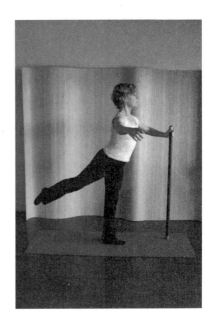

3

4

Exercise #16 (Standing Pilates): 4-Way Leg Flow

Resources

BOOK

Standing Pilates: Strengthen and Tone Your Body Wherever You Are
> By Joan Breibart

DVDs

Do More Pilates STANDING
> With Niece Pecenka and Bea Wood

Fletcher Pilates® Towelwork DVD
> From Balanced Body

Standing Pilates
> From Yuu Fujita & The PhysicalMind Institute

The Method - Standing Pilates Blend
> By Katalin Zamiar

Susan Tuttle's In Home Fitness: Standing Pilates
> By Susan Tuttle

ONLINE COURSE

Evolution 201: Matwork, Standing & Circular Pilates
> From The PhysicalMind Institute

ONLINE VIDEO (using TheMethod Pilates' Tye4®)

Tye4® & Standing Pilates
> Viewable at: http://www.youtube.com/watch?v=BrIrrMALQEU

Chapter 7: Circular Work

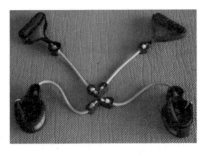

Circular Pilates™ is a clever expansion of the PhysicalMind (PMI)'s trainings. It was introduced by Joan Breibart as the Initiation 301 course. It is a very pleasing and three dimensional expansion of earlier standing work, which was developed in collaboration with Marika Molnar, a Physical Therapist and PMI's Clinical Advisor. It was originally conceived as an evolutionary concept that added rotational exercises of great value to aging students who were just beginning to practice Pilates' exercises.

Evolving Pilates' Greek Mind-Body Connection

Expanding Pilates' repertoire beyond simple linear movements, Breibart's Circular Pilates™ program offers rotational and 3-dimensional space usage, as well as larger body movements. In practice, these movements engage the brain in a broader manner, employing cues that emphasize what is called the "Brain Connector Fundamental". In this training, limb movements are also synchronized to enhance the mind-body connection through the sometimes complex movement paths, and even involving eye tracking to facilitate brain engagement.

Benefits of Circular Exercises

Teachers understand that people injure themselves when they perform everyday tasks such as parallel parking their car, or lifting and reaching movements that are followed by twisting. Many people are weak during rotational movements. They have difficulties safely connecting upper body movements with lower body movements. Pilates-inspired circular movements address these problems while building strength and simultaneously improving coordination and balance. Instructors can teach such exercises, while continuously moving at regular or half time speeds, to enhance concentration.

Overall, the Circular Pilates™ repertoire offers students (and teachers) a challenging and engaging series of movements that stimulate balancing and proprioceptive awareness. In particular, as instructors that have taught such classes to older populations, these exercises are indeed effective, challenging and fun.

Pose #1: Preparatory position

Stand relaxed and balanced with feet together.

Pose #2: Lifting one leg

While slowly inhaling to a count of four, lift your left knee and raise both arms to the horizontal and out towards the sides.

Pose #3: Twisting toward the lifted leg

Slowly exhale to a count of four while twisting your arms, head and torso to the left. Let your eyes follow the movement.

Pose #4: Raising the arms and finishing

- While slowly inhaling to a count of four, extend the left leg forward while raising the arms upwards.
- Complete the exercise by exhaling slowly to a count of four, untwisting the body and returning the leg and arms back to the starting position of pose 1 above.

Tips

Move your head in line with your torso. Keep your hips even and facing front.

Repetitions

Repeat six times per side before repeating poses 1 to 4 with the other leg. As you become stronger, you can increase the repetitions from six to eight or ten.

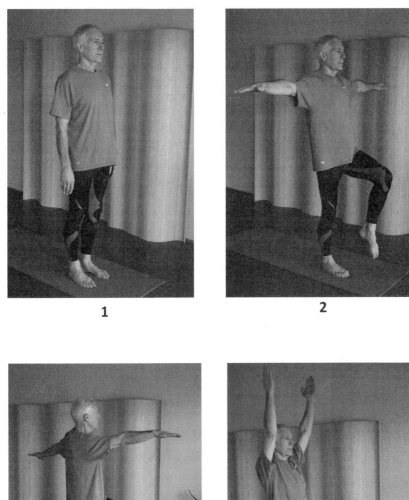

1

2

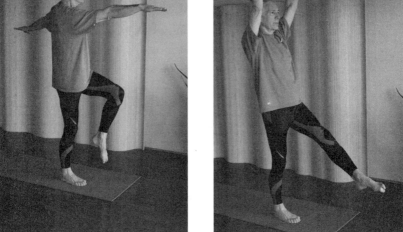

3

4

Exercise #17 (Circular Pilates): One Legged Lift w/Balance Twist

Pose #1: Preparatory position

Sit comfortably with legs in parallel position and arms outwards.

Pose #2: Oblique roll down

Slowly exhale to a count of four while spiraling your arms, head and torso to the right and down. Place your right palm on the floor behind you and to the right. Draw your abdominals inward and upward as you slide your right arm down the diagonal. Curl your tailbone underneath you while continuing your exhalation, completing your roll down to the floor along this right, rear diagonal path.

Pose #3: Circling to other side

Continue moving smoothly while performing these remaining elements:

- Draw your left arm upwards and overhead, and then lower it toward your other arm and hand.
- Slowly begin to inhale to a count of four while untwisting your torso away from the right diagonal. Allow your left arm to now circle past the front of your face while rolling your torso toward the left side. Move your head in the same rolling fashion as the arm, following the motion of your left arm with your eyes.
- Follow these movements of left arm, head and torso by drawing your right arm across your body while rolling your torso to the left side. Continue circularly with the right arm, with your left palm on the ground and right arm moving now forwards along the same diagonal as your left arm.

Pose #4: Oblique roll up

Press down with your left palm, grounding the left side of your hips against the mat. Begin a smooth exhalation to a count of four while reaching outwards and forwards with your right fingers and arm. Roll up obliquely back to pose 1. Reverse poses 1 - 4 in the other direction.

Tips

As you become more comfortable with the three dimensional complexity of this exercise, you can extend your exhalation duration from a count of four to longer counts of six or eight in poses 2 and 4.

Repetitions

Start with four. Increase to six or eight as you become stronger.

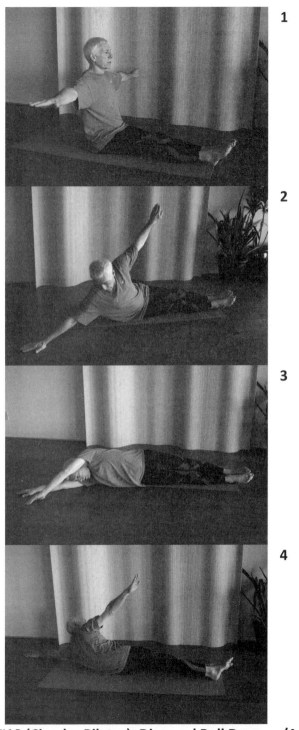

Exercise #18 (Circular Pilates): Diagonal Roll Down w/Arm Reach

Resources

ONLINE COURSE

Evolution 201: Matwork, Standing & Circular Pilates

Course Info and Video Excerpt from The PhysicalMind Institute:
http://themethodpilates.com/matwork/evolution-201/

ONLINE VIDEOs

Standing and Circular Pilates using the Tye4® (from TheMethod Pilates)
Viewable at: http://www.youtube.com/watch?v=BrIrrMALQEU

Fundamental Pilates Movements with Circularity
Viewable at: http://www.youtube.com/watch?v=oo7xovCXajs

ONLINE PDF (from the PhysicalMind Institute)

http://www.themethodpilates.com/items/pdf/circular_pilates.pdf

Chapter 8: Unstable Surfaces

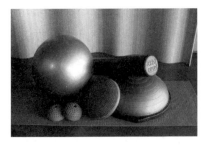 Pilates' instructors use unstable surfaces as props because they force the students to pay more attention to their bodies to maintain alignment and balance. Using these sorts of props is very effective in developing a student's awareness of their body in space, called *proprioception* by physical therapists.

Although we demonstrate sample exercises in this chapter with a foam roller, and exercise stones (hard rubber half-domes), there are many other examples of unstable props. You may encounter large Swiss balls, the small balls seen earlier in Chapter 4, balance beams and discs, and specialized, registered props like the **BOSU®** lateral dome.

Why Do Unstable Surfaces Enhance Pilates' Exercises?

Each unstable prop variation forces the proprioceptors in the deep stabilizing muscles in the spine and torso to fire. This proprioception enhances the coordination of muscles, bones, tendons, and joints without having to actually look at the body parts that you are coordinating in either a daily activity or complex exercise. The net result is that you develop improved body awareness. Your body is forced to provide needed extra support by activating deep core muscles, promoting both balance and alignment.

Emphasize Stabilization First

Establishing stability before attempting mobility, balance and coordination is paramount to success and safety when using unstable surfaces. Each piece of equipment in this arena reflects a simple design and can be adapted to a variety of techniques that enhance balance, body awareness, muscle recruitment, strengthening and mobilization of the spine and multiple other body parts. A qualified instructor ensures that you work in many different positions and circumstances that reflect common movements from daily life.

Instructions for One Legged Circles on Foam Roller

Pose #1: Preparatory position

Lie lengthwise along the roller with palms pressed against the ground on both sides of your foam roller. The left knee is bent with sole of the foot against the floor. The right leg is bent in tabletop position. Begin a slow inhalation to straighten the right leg upwards into pose 2.

Pose #2: Begin the circle

Continue inhaling to a count of four as the right leg circles outward to the right and downwards towards the left leg.

Pose #3: Continue the circle

Continue the circle in space. At the halfway point, finish your inhalation and begin a slow exhalation that will last through poses 3 and 4.

Pose #4: Finish strongly

- Finish your exhalation as you consciously draw the right leg circularly back to perpendicular (pose 2), lifting your abs upwards toward your ribs and hollowing your belly.
- Repeat poses 2, 3 and 4 four times in one direction before switching to four times in the other circular direction. This constitutes one series for one leg. Repeat the dual directional series on the other leg to constitute one complete repetition.

Tips (and challenges)

Challenge opportunities abound with unstable surfaces. Any one or more of these will focus your balancing efforts further into your core musculature:

- You can extend the non-traveling leg (the one with the bent knee in the pictures) into a straight position.
- You can also enlarge the circle that your leg traces in space to place additional challenge on your abs.
- During the second half of each circle, while drawing the leg back to the starting position, speed up the movement of the leg.
- Even further, you can lift one or both of your palms off the ground while performing the one legged circles.

Repetitions

Perform each complete repetition twice, with both legs. As you become stronger, increase the overall repetitions from two to four or six.

234

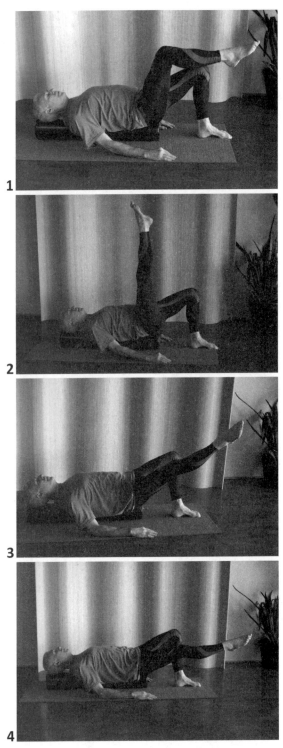

Exercise #19 (Unstable): One Legged Circles on Foam Roller

Pose #1: Preparatory sense of balance

Begin on hands and knees, gaining a sense of balance on the half spheres ('stones'). If this feels too unstable, remove the stones from the rear knees. Perhaps, you might only use one stone under one forward hand as well. Align your arms vertically with palms directly under shoulders. Align your upper legs vertically so your knees are directly underneath your hips.

Pose #2: Spinal balance position

Inhale slowly to a count of four while raising your left arm and right leg upwards to align in parallel with the mat. Reach forwards, extending your arm all the way to your fingertips. Similarly, extend your rear leg backwards, lengthening all the way through the leg to the toes.

Pose #3: Opposite knee to elbow

Exhale slowly to a count of four, moving into a cat stretch and hollowing the belly, while drawing your right knee forwards and slightly inwards. Simultaneously, bend and draw your right elbow backwards toward the left knee. Adjust your breath so that you smoothly move the arm and leg toward each other through the entire span of the exhalation.

Pose #4: Restabilize in spinal balance

Reverse this pose 3 by extending the knee and elbow away from each other to return to the spinal balance seen in pose 2. Repeat with the same knee-leg combination for 4-6 times before switching to the other knee-leg combination.

Tips

If you do not have this particular prop, you can still perform this exercise without any prop at all. Alternatively, with one or two mini balls, you can place one or both balls under the forward hand(s) for a challenging balance.

Repetitions

Repeat the exercise (poses 2, 3 and 4) four times. As you become stronger, you can increase the repetitions from four to six.

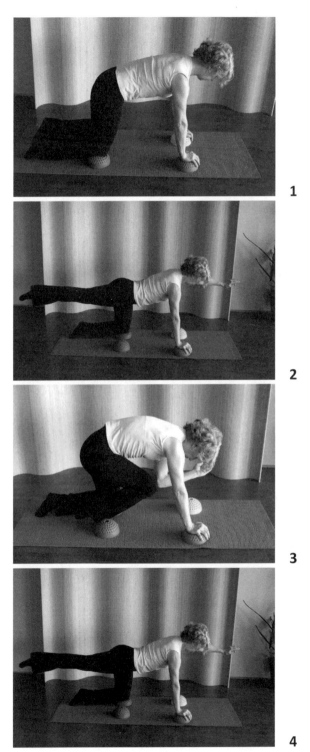

1

2

3

4

Exercise #20 (Unstable): Spinal Balance w/Knee to Elbow

Resources

BOOKs

Foam Roller Workbook: Illustrated Step-by-Step Guide to Stretching, Strengthening and Rehabilitative Techniques
     by Karl Knopf M.D.

Pilates: Using Small Props for Big Results
     By Christine Romani-Ruby

Get On It!: BOSU Balance Trainer Workouts
     by Jane Aronovitch, Miriane Taylor, and Colleen Craig

DVDs

STOTT PILATES - Stability Ball Challenge
     With Moira Merrithew & PJ O'Clair

STOTT PILATES: Essential BOSU and Intermediate BOSU (2 separate DVDs)
     With Moira Merrithew

Power Systems Pilates Foam Roller Workout DVD
     By Power Systems

OPTP Pilates Foam Roller Workout DVD
     From OPTP

STOTT PILATES: Foam Roller Challenge
     By Moira Merrithew

Chapter 9: Fusion Classes

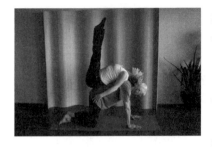 Some students and instructors confess to getting high on multitasking, or more specifically, blending more than simply Pilates exercises themselves into a workout. Pilates himself emphasized the simultaneity of strengthening muscles on one side of the body while stretching other muscles on the reverse side of the body.

Evolving this instructional awareness in the 21st Century has seen an evolution of blended approaches that merge Pilates' exercises in creative ways into expanded arenas.

Fusion Can Be Multi-disciplinary, Multi-prop, or Multi-person

Yogilates® from Jonathan Urla in Pennsylvania merges yoga with Pilates. A growing number of other instructors are now creating and offering novel Partner Pilates exercises and classes that coordinate two exercisers in back-to-back or feet-to-feet positions. Whereas Pilates' exercises appealed to many dancers in the early 20th Century, current dancers are merging Pilates with well-known dance movements.

Jillian Hessel is a former dancer and, as a Pilates professional, notes that both disciplines stress excellence of movement. The goal of both dance and Pilates' work is effortlessness and flowing movement. Dance can be aesthetic and so can the results of Pilates' exercise. Combining the two is a natural for a fusion class, and can naturally lead to both ease and grace in everyday life.

Commonality Seen in the Fusion

Other combination classes arise from the ingenuity of instructors around the world. A growing number of instructors are developing merged discipline classes between Pilates and aquatics, Pilates and boxing, Pilates and other martial arts, such as tai chi, karate, and chi gung.

Key elements are common to all of these merging disciplines. Each seeks to stimulate greater awareness and balance in a developing body. Each requires a strong core and movements that originate from that core with strength and grace extending outwards to the limbs.

Pose #21A: Back to back preparation for spine twist

Sit up tall, directly on your sitz bones, and back to back with your partner. Draw your abdomens inward and toward each other while reaching your arms outwards to the sides. For an extra stretch, you could draw your toes backward, flexing your feet.

Pose #21B: Spine twist, each way

Relaxing your shoulders and ribs downwards, slowly exhale while twisting your bodies to your right sides. Maintain connection to each other. Inhale to a count of four to return to the position seen in pose 1; repeat all instructions to your left sides.

Pose #22A: Feet to feet preparation for single leg stretch

Lie on your backs in tabletop position. Your feet should be flexed with the soles of the feet against your partners'. Inhale to a count of four to begin.

Pose #22B: Single leg stretch, each leg

a. Exhale slowly to a count of four while each of you floats your head and shoulders upwards, extends your right leg and bends your left knee towards the chest.

b. Place your left hand for alignment just to the left of your ankle.

c. Place your right hand just below the left knee, using the hand to gently draw the bent leg toward you for an extra hip stretch on that leg.

d. Inhale to the same count of four while reversing the legs, as well as the positioning of your hands at and on the other leg.

e. Repeat instruction *c* and *d* a total of four times. Return to figure 22A.

f. Reverse sides by repeating instructions *a-e*, this time starting with the exhalation and extension of the left leg.

Tips

If your hamstrings are tight in exercise 21, you can sit on a pillow or blanket to align your backs better.

Repetitions

Repeat the exercise to each side (21A-B) or with each leg (22A-B) four times. As you become stronger and more flexible, you can increase the overall repetitions from four to six or eight.

240

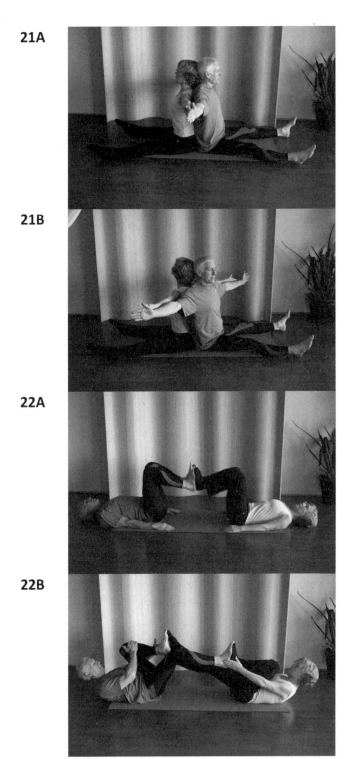

21A

21B

22A

22B

Exercise #21-22 (Partner): Spine twists & Single leg stretches

Pose #1: Preparatory position

Begin standing with your feet in a slight or full *turn out* position. Hold a prop (stick or taut towel, tube, or strap) down at about thigh level.

Pose #2: Lifting

Inhale slowly to a count of four while lifting your right leg outwards and off the mat, balancing on your left leg and lifting the arms and prop overhead. Toes of both feet are pointed outwards.

Pose #3: Bending

Exhale slowly to a count of four, lowering and bending the right knee into a side lunge. Simultaneously, bend (laterally flex) the upper body toward the right side. Maintain spacing and centeredness of the head to the arms and prop.

Pose #4: Finishing

Inhale slowly to a count of four while lifting the upper body and prop back to center. At the same time, lift the knee of the right leg back up into a centered and balanced position in front. Your weight is now balanced on the left leg. Slowly lower the right leg, and both arms, while exhaling to a count of four and returning to pose 1. Reverse the sequence of poses 2, 3 and 4 to the other side, starting with a lift of your left leg.

Tips

As you learn this sequencing, and become stronger, you can pick up the pace to make this a faster, more dynamic exercise.

Repetitions

Repeat four times to each side before moving on to another exercise. As you become stronger, you can increase the repetitions from four to six or eight twelve.

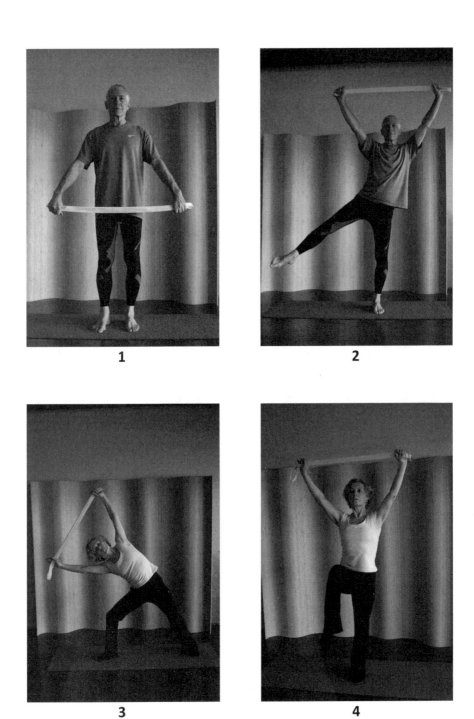

1

2

3

4

Exercise #23 (Bar/Towel/Strap/Ball Fusion): Side Bend

Resources

BOOKs

Yoga and Pilates for Everyone
        By Freedman, Gibbs, Hall, Kelly, Monks, and Smith

Jennifer Kries' Pilates Plus Method: The Unique Combination of Yoga, Dance, and Pilates
        By Jennifer Kries

STOTT PILATES: Intense Sculpting Challenge
        By Moira Merrithew

Yogilates®: Integrating Yoga and Pilates for Complete Fitness, Strength, and Flexibility
        By Jonathan Urla

DVDs

Yogilates – Beginner, Intermediate and Advanced Workouts (Separate DVDs)
        By Jonathan Urla

Attitude Ballet and Pilates Fusion
        From Bernadette Giorgi

Piloxing
        By Viveca Jensen

Water Pilates Dvd & Instructional Cd
        By Carol Argo

The Method - Pilates Fusion - A Ballet & Pilates Dance Blend (2006)
        By Katalin Zamiar

Chapter 10: Sports Specific Pilates

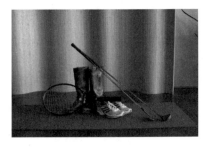 There has been a veritable explosion of novel mergers between basic Pilates' techniques and sport-specific applications. Just to list a few, we've seen the development of Pilates' classes and programs for equestrians, swimmers, golfers, tennis players, cyclists, runners, skiers, and even NFL players.

All of these programs draw on careful breath work and mind-body coordination discussed in Part I (Your Health) of this book, as well as the six fundamental principles of Pilates' original exercises that were discussed in Part II (Contrology) of this book. All sports require their own blend of core strength, spinal and torsional flexibility, shoulder girdle, arm, and leg strengthening, and overall body awareness, balance, and proprioception.

Fundamental Pilates' Benefits for Equestrians

By now, you realize that Pilates' exercises not only improve body awareness but equally well enhance flexibility, balance, and strength. This benefits equestrians in a variety of ways, all of which add up to more enjoyable and controlled experiences for both horse and rider. Specifically, Pilates' work helps by lengthening the spine and strengthening the core, which in turn stabilizes your body during all equestrian movements. Increasing flexibility, strength, and balance helps riders to create a deeper seat. Simultaneously, this aids in enhancing your lower back's suppleness and potentially increasing hip independence.

Equestrian Benefits of Increased Flexibility and a Stronger Core

Horseback riders will develop a stable lower body and core base from Pilates' work. This results in freer and smoother movement of arms and legs. This leads to clearer aids when cueing your horse, as well as improved ability to hold jumping form, if you are at that level. All riders will discover that they maintain better overall posture and stay more comfortable both during and after rides. Improved posture through Pilates directly results in easier maintenance of a neutral pelvis, better absorption of a horse's movement, and better coordination of your body with that of your horse. Equestrians who have applied Pilates' techniques to their riding have reported a closer feel, and a more trusting riding relationship with their horse. As occasional riders, we know that the goal of a more responsive and confident horse is only a few more Pilates' exercises away.

Pilates for Swimmers

Swimming obviously demands a strong core, which Pilates directly develops. The direct result of Pilates' work is that a swimmer is more able to maintain their scapula, shoulders, pelvis and spine in a balanced and aligned fashion. This allows a swimmer to lift their arms up and out of the water without straining the neck muscles; this leads to less overall wear and tear on the body and a faster swim. The core muscles used in swimming emphasize the deeper transverse abdominals. The strengthening of these muscles is a major result of well executed Pilates' movements. Pilates' techniques such as slow and controlled motion, focus, and alignment also bear directly on improved swimming.

Benefits of Pilates for Swimmers

Pilates and swimming are a great combination for swimmers of all ages. The aspect of balance that is so crucial to swimmers is an obvious and direct connector of the two. Although Pilates does not offer the potential cardio benefits of swimming, the controlled gentleness of Pilates' exercises, when coupled with swimming, is a wonderful approach to whole body wellness, as well as an often recommended dual combination for both wellness and rehabilitation.

Swimmers who have taken Pilates' classes have reported that the emphases on core strength, alignment, and posture translate directly to movement, positioning, and faster speeds in the water. Pilates further helps by encouraging correct breathing patterns that are synchronized with movements both in and out of water. Six-time Olympic coach and Head Coach of Stanford Women's Swim Team, Richard Quick, made Pilates a standard part of his Swim Team's training program.

The net effect of improving core strength with Pilates is that you will naturally depend less on arm strength and more on a balanced use of your entire body for swimming strokes. Long distance swimmers report increased endurance as a result of this coordination of arm and leg movements with the core, plus the extension of energy from the abs to the extremities. Beyond this, Pilates improves flexibility and coordination, which naturally leads to reduced risk of injury and improvement of fundamental swimming strokes.

Pilates for Golfers

Pilates and golf share similar core principles and both offer mind-body conditioning. Pilates taught symmetrical and coordinated movements that lead to increased range of motion. Golfers gain enhanced balance and fluid motion from Pilates' work, as well as specifically improved core and hip stability, flexibility, a wider range-of-motion, and more effective breathing patterns. Pilates' exercises specifically help golfers to achieve power, precision, and fluid motion in every swing. This is due to the coordinated, sequential muscle-firing for deep stabilizers, hip flexors and extensors, hip abductors and adductors, as well as spinal flexors, extensors and rotators.

Benefits of Pilates for Golfers

Pilates' training strengthens the back, resulting in increased core stability. It also improves balance during an increased rotational range of motion. The result is that you will be able to hit deeper and straighter balls.

Yes, your golf pro can improve your technique by changing your stance, grip or hip turn ratio. But your body underlies all faults, and causes a great many of them. Retraining your body through Pilates can improve the fundamentals of your ability to swing the club, while preventing injuries and increasing overall performance. Pilates also offers a wealth of exercises that can correct existing physical limitations in golfers. These limitations include lack of flexibility, lack of core strength, limited rotation, instability of hips or shoulders, weakness in hips, legs, wrist or forearms, and total body strength asymmetry.

Pilates for Runners

Pilates' exercises are replete with graceful, flowing movements. They build strength without bulking up muscles. They are naturally attractive to runners, many of whom have noted both increased flexibility and strength, plus reduced muscle soreness in legs and knees, after adopting a Pilates-based training regimen.

Benefits of Pilates for Runners

Runners soon realize that Pilates offers not only strength enhancements but an effective, progressive stretching routine as well. Well designed Pilates exercises stretch muscles that runners need stretched and that might otherwise slow them down or lead to serious injuries. Many exercises focus on torso stretching during abdominal strengthening, both helping to warm up the core muscles and stretch the intercostal muscles that connect the ribs.

Related to the intercostals, Pilates emphasizes terrific breathing skills. Flexible intercostals make breathing easier and smoother and can improve lung capacity.

Pilates for All Sports

The focus on breathing in Pilates helps all sports endeavors. Efficient and careful application of Pilates' fundamentals and exercises strengthens and stretches muscles. Movements are better coordinated. Breathing is improved. You will quickly observe improvements in any sport or physical activity that you pursue. Muscles that were previously sore after sport may be so for shorter periods of time, or not at all.

Active sports endure a variety of impacts, whether to the legs, arms or other body parts. Soccer players are subjected to constant impact when running, as are runners. Tennis players and players of other racquet sports are subjected to the same rotational torques and strain that golfers experience. The various ground forces at each step travel up from the legs to the lower back and rib cage. Core strength developed through Pilates enables your entire body to better deal with, cushion, and resist the impact. With improved body alignment and balance, every sports practitioner will be able to more efficiently redistribute forces throughout the body. The overall result is more endurance, less fatigue, and less pain.

Resources

BOOKs

A Gymnastic Riding System Using Mind, Body, and Spirit: Progressive Training for Rider and Horse
    By Betsy Steiner with Jennifer Bryant

The Golfer's Guide to Pilates: Step-by-Step Exercises to Strengthen Your Game
    By Monica Clyde

Pilates for the Outdoor Athlete
    By Lauri Stricker

The Complete Guide to Joseph H. Pilates' Techniques of Physical Conditioning: With Special Help for Back Pain and Sports Training
    By Alan Menezes

The Anatomy of Exercise and Movement for the Study of Dance, Pilates, Sports, and Yoga
    By Jo Ann Staugaard-Jones

Sports Pilates: How to Prevent and Overcome Sports Injuries
    By Paul Massey

DVDs

Swimalates: Pilates for Swimmers (DVD)
    by June Quick

Hole in One Pilates DVD
    by Hole In One (Available at Amazon.com)

Pilates for Golf (2 DVDs)
    From Stott Pilates

Appendix A: Glossary

Abs:
Refers to the four stabilizing muscles (rectus abdominis, external oblique, internal oblique, and transverse abdominis) that form a girdle spanning from the front of the torso to the back, up to the ribs and down to the pelvis.

Abduction:
Muscle contraction that draws a limb away from the midline of the body.

Adduction:
A muscle contraction that draws a limb closer to the midline of the body.

Anterior:
Toward the front of the body.

Articulation:
Moving the joints of the body; also, moving the spinal column one vertebra at a time.

Bilateral:
A movement with both sides of the body.

Breathing:
One of the six fundamental principles of Pilates work: coordinating a full inhalation and exhalation in concert with each exercise is paramount to effective Pilates work.

Centering:
A second one of the six fundamental principles of Pilates work: a conscious focus on beginning each exercise from the core (central) part of the muscular body.

Cervical Vertebrae:
The seven vertebrae located in the neck.

Concentration:
A third one of the six fundamental principles of Pilates work: paying close attention to the elements of each exercise for maximum benefit.

Concentric muscle contraction:
Muscular shortening during contraction.

Control:
A fourth one of the six fundamental principles of Pilates work: each exercise requires complete, constant, and consistent muscular control.

Contrology:
Joseph Pilates' original name for his total program of exercise. 'Pilates' has replaced Contrology for the total program of exercises, both Pilates' original 34 exercises, and all evolutionary extensions of his program.

250

Core:
The complete, three dimensional set of all the bones, joints and muscles in the center of the body, working together to stabilize the body and mobilize movement.

Eccentric muscle contraction:
Muscle lengthening while contracting.

Extension:
Increasing the angle between two bones, and the movement of a joint which increases the joint angle.

First-generation teacher:
Refers to any teacher of Pilates who learned the Method directly under Joseph Pilates himself.

Flexion:
Joint movement that decreases the joint angle.

Flow:
A fifth one of the six fundamental principles of Pilates work: smooth and fluid movement is encouraged during the movements associated with each Pilates exercise.

Functional Fitness:
Refers to fitness exercises that enhance the same kind of movements performed during everyday activities.

Hip Flexors:
Central muscles around the hips; responsible for flexing the upper legs.

Hundred:
The first of Pilates' original exercises; used to warm up the muscles and promote oxygenation and blood flow.

Hyperextension:
Undesirable and unhealthy joint movement beyond the normal anatomical position. Sometimes referred to as locked elbow or knee.

Imprinting:
Refers to isolating the individual vertebra of the spine during Pilates' exercises.

Intercostal muscles:
Muscles that lie diagonally between ribs, and assist in controlling expansion and contraction of your rib cage when you breathe.

Isometric Contraction:
Muscle contraction, generally while holding a position, that does not change the muscle's length.

Joseph Pilates:
Born December 9, 1883 – Died October 9, 1967. The developer of the Pilates' Contrology method of physical fitness.

Ligament:
Connective tissue between bone and bone.
Lumbar Vertebrae:
The five vertebrae located in the lower back.
Magic Circle:
An isometric ring that consists of a flexible circle with handles.
Mat/Matwork:
A mat is the rubbery, thin, and solid sheet of material used to lie on during Pilates' exercises. Matwork refers to exercises performed on a mat.
Medial:
Related to or moving toward the midline of the body.
Modifications:
Variations in an exercise, offered for appropriateness to either body type or experience with Pilates exercises.
Navel to spine:
A cueing guideline during Pilates exercises; suggests the stabilizing effort of drawing your abdominal muscles up while imagining your navel being drawn closer to your spine.
Neutral pelvis:
A natural and relaxed positioning of the pelvis; not tucked under, not arched back, and not tilted to either side.
Neutral spine:
A normal and natural position of the back that maintains the natural curves of the cervical, thoracic, and lumbar vertebrae.
Pelvis:
Portion of the body that is comprised of the hip bones, sacrum, and coccyx.
Pilates Principles:
The six fundamental principles governing the effective execution of Pilates exercises --- Breathing, Centering, Control, Concentration, Flow, and Precision.
Posterior:
Referring to the back surface of the body.
Powerhouse:
Refers to the entire set of muscles in the center of your body, including the abdominals, back, pelvic floor, and gluteals.
Precision:
A third one of the six fundamental principles of Pilates work: each individual portion of each exercise must be executed exactly according to exercise design.

Proprioception:
The sense of the relative positioning of connected parts of the body and of the effort needed during movements.

Prone:
A lengthwise position of the body, facing downwards toward the mat.

Scooping your abs:
Drawing the abdominal muscles both upwards and inwards while stabilizing the body and supporting the back.

Percussive Breathing:
Quick in-and-out breathing patterns used in conjunction with precise exercise movements. Developed by Ron Fletcher to sequentially breathe in multiple times through your nose, and then blow out successively multiple times through the mouth.

Sitz Bones:
The bony parts that one feels when you sit on any firm surface. They are actually bony landmarks of the pelvic girdle and are technically known as *the Ischial Tuberosities.* Alternatively called *sits bones* or *sit bones*.

Spine:
Consisting of twenty-four vertebrae, and sometimes called the vertebral column, it consists of seven cervical, twelve thoracic, five lumbar, 4-5 fused sacral, and 3-4 fused coccyx vertebrae.

Supine:
A lengthwise positioning in which you are lying on your back.

Tabletop Legs:
A positioning of the legs in which the knees are bent, the thighs are perpendicular to the floor, and the shins are parallel to the floor.

Tendon:
Tissue that connects bone to muscle.

Thoracic Vertebrae:
The twelve vertebrae located in the upper and mid back.

Unilateral:
An exercise movement that uses a limb on one side of the body while trying to stabilize the rest of the body.

Vertebrae:
The 32 to 34 small bones that make up the spine. Intervertebral discs provide cushioning between the vertebrae as well as allowing elastic movement of the entire back and spine.

Zipper:
An instructional image for drawing the lower abs up and in, as in zipping up a coat.

Appendix B: Index

abs, abdominals, **234**, **246**, **253**

Articulation, **250**

beds and chairs, **71**

Black, Madeline, **187**

breathing, **4**, **11**, **57-60**, **83**, **96**, **101-102**, **218**, **246-248**, **253**

Breathing, **83**, **102**, **248**, **250-253**

Breibart, Joan, **186-187**, **221**, **226-227**

Centering, **83**, **221**, **250**, **252**

Circular Pilates, **186**, **226-227**, **229**, **231-232**

Common Sense Remedies, **44**

Concentration, **83**, **250**, **252**

Control, **7**, **83-84**, **93**, **179**, **190**, **250**, **252**

Contrology, **5-7**, **11-12**, **15-16**, **25**, **35**, **36**, **52–55**, **57**, **81-85**, **87**, **90**, **93**, **95**, **98-112**, **186**, **245**, **250-251**

core, **11**, **83**, **186**, **189**, **191**, **197**, **209**, **215**, **221**, **233-234**, **239**, **245-247**, **250**

Endelman, Ken, **187**

equestrian, **245**

Exercises

21st Century, **4–5**

Biceps, **217**

Boomerang, **7**, **93**, **170**, **171**

chest expansion, **222**, **223**

Cork-Screw, **7**, **93**, **132**, **133**

Criss-Cross, **212**, **213**

Diagonal Roll Down, **231**

Double Leg Stretch, **7**, **93**, **126**, **127**, **198**, **199**

Hip Twist, **7**, **93**, **158**, **159**

Leg-Pull, **7**, **93**, **162**, **163**, **164**, **165**

Magic Circle - Biceps, **192**, **198- 199**

Magic Circle - Chest Press, **192**

Magic Circle - Lat Press, **192**

Magic Circle - Rainbow, **194-195**

Magic Circle - Mid-Back, **192**

One leg circle, **7**, **93**, **120**, **121**

Rocking, **7**, **93**, **176**, **177**

Roll Up, **7**, **93**, **116-117**

Roll-Over, **7**, **93**, **118**, **119**

Saw, **7**, **93**, **134**, **135**, **203**

Scissors, **7**, **93**, **144**, **145**

Side Bend, **7**, **93**, **168**, **169**, **242**, **243**

Spinal Balance w/Knee to Elbow, **236**, **237**

Spine Stretch, **7**, **93**, **128**, **129**, **203**

Spine Twist, **7**, **93**, **150**, **151**

Swan, **7**, **93**, **136**, **137**, **206**, **207**

The Hundred, **7**, **93**, **114-115**, **205**, **251**

Fletcher, Ron, **186-187, 221, 253**

Flow, **83, 196, 224, 225, 251, 252**

Gallagher, Sean, **187**

golf, **247**

Kryzanowska, Romana, 186-**188, 191**

Larkam, Elizabeth, **187**

Merrithew, Moira, *See* Stott

Magic Circle, **191–96**

mind-body connection, **39, 56**

neutral spine, pelvis, **186, 198, 245**

Percussive breathing, **253**

PhysicalMind Institute, **4, 187, 190, 221, 226, 232**

posture, **32, 64–70**

powerhouse', **83, 191**

Precision, **83, 84, 252**

Principles, **5, 35, 36, 44, 49, 54-57, 65, 68, 78, 82-84, 110, 188, 197, 245, 247, 250-252**

Runners, **247**

sports, **16, 19, 25, 84, 103, 245, 248**

Standing Pilates, **186, 221, 223, 225, 226**

Stott, Moira, **186, 214, 220, 249**

Swimming, **7, 93, 160-161, 246**

Urla, Jonathan **239, 244**

Vertebra, **102, 105**

vertebrae, **68, 105, 252-253**

Yogilates® **239, 244**

Yoga, **202, 244, 249**

Zipper, **253**

Pilates Blog and Private Workshops
From Presentation Dynamics LLC

See our well known Pilates Blog at:
http://JosephPilates.org
for links to Pilates' original books
and the latest evolutionary expansion
of Joseph Pilates' ground breaking trainings.

Private Workshops are also available at your location
Send an inquiry email to
admin@presentation-dynamics.net